Surgical
Decision Making

Surgical
Decision Making

F. T. de Dombal
Director of the Clinical Information Science Unit, the University of Leeds and Hon. Consultant Surgeon, St James (University) Hospital, Leeds

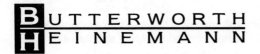

Butterworth-Heinemann Ltd
Linacre House, Jordan Hill, Oxford OX2 8DP

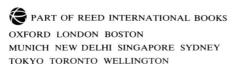 PART OF REED INTERNATIONAL BOOKS

OXFORD LONDON BOSTON
MUNICH NEW DELHI SINGAPORE SYDNEY
TOKYO TORONTO WELLINGTON

First published 1993

© Butterworth-Heinemann Ltd 1993

British Library Cataloguing in Publication Data
Dombal, F. T. De
  Surgical Decision Making
  I. Title
  617

ISBN 0 7506 0704 1

Library of Congress Cataloguing in Publication Data
De Dombal, F. T.
  Surgical decision making/F.T. de Dombal.
  p.   cm.
  Includes bibliographical references and index.
  ISBN 0 7506 0704 1
  1. Surgery–Decision making.   I. Title
  [DNLM: 1. Decision Making.   2. Diagnosis, Surgical–methods.   WO
  141 D299s]
  RD31.5.D43   1993
  617–dc20
                                                        92–49547
                                                        CIP
Typeset in 11 on 12pt Times Roman by TecSet Ltd, Wallington, Surrey
Printed and bound in Great Britain by Biddles Ltd, Guildford and King's
Lynn

Contents

Preface

The basic idea behind the book is simple. Clinical medical students are not taught to make decisions. They are not taught to manage situations. They learn these skills the hard way, often with great difficulty, only after qualification. Should a student be perceptive enough to realize this and look for help in the textbooks or the literature, the student is confronted with a treatise (often abusive about the medical profession) in which every other paragraph contains a mathematical equation.

This small book aims to fill the gap by presenting some of the issues to clinical students, junior surgeons and others in such a way that they can concentrate upon issues rather than mathematics, practical problems rather than theoretical obscurities, and differential diagnoses rather than differential equations. Hopefully, in this way the reader will receive some practical guidance, before the reader is in a situation that requires immediate attention at 3 a.m. after 30 min sleep!

Although this is a small book, its gestation period has occupied over a quarter of a century. Back in the mid 1960s, when I was a senior registrar and resident surgical officer in a large busy teaching hospital (the General Infirmary at Leeds), I began to wonder why I only got 70% of my acute cases right as regards initial diagnosis, why I found it increasingly difficult to keep up even with one specialized field (inflammatory bowel disease), and, most of all, why the students increasingly became glassy-eyed when I bestowed upon them the benefits of my encyclopaedic knowledge of surgery! In conversation with other senior registrars, I was surprised but somewhat relieved to find that they encountered similar difficulties; and in 1969 the Medical Research

Council was kind enough to provide me with the (then huge) sum of around £10 000 to study human and computer aided diagnosis.

Since that time much has changed. The Clinical Information Science Unit, which I now direct, has published literally hundreds of studies concerning decision support, diagnosis, human and computer performance – and we now have a much better idea of the strengths and weaknesses of both. Far more important, however, the world around us has changed. The medical curriculum has become increasingly crowded with fact after fact after fact, and students increasingly have difficulty in taking in all of this. Sadly, because student numbers have increased dramatically, while patient turnover in hospital has speeded up, access to patients has decreased, as has direct experience of observing clinical care at first hand.

In the last few years a number of calls have gone out for a change of emphasis with less factual learning and more problem solving in the medical curriculum. I concur thoroughly, but the problem is that no one has any evidence or experience as to how this can be done. Well almost no one, because informally in the 1970s and 1980s and now more regularly, I have taught surgical decision making to students in their first clinical year as part of their routine course. The feedback from those students who eventually qualify has been in general favourable, and indeed sometimes quite gratifying, often along the lines that the course has helped them when a year or two later they were left alone to cope on the surgical wards.

This type of response is really what made me accept, when approached and asked to write a short text on surgical decision making. I have neither the scientific wisdom nor the mathematical firepower to provide a definitive treatise on some of the aspects now in fashion (e.g. chaos theory, neural networks, and so on), but there may well be a place for an expanded version of the lecture notes to the course, which might hopefully appeal to clinical medical students and also newly qualified surgeons.

This approach has rather dictated the style of the book. You will find that it is written in simple and conversational style. This is deliberate. There are quite a number of learned scientific mathematical treatises on decision making. The problem is that medical students will not read them. What I have tried to write instead is a conversational version in the hope that this introduction will allow medical students and young surgeons to understand what is happening in the world of decision making – and for those who become interested as I did there are other more erudite volumes to which they can progress!

As a result of this approach, you will find few formulae and few references to learned journals in the book. Both exist (in profusion!) in the textbooks and the literature, but I firmly believe that clinical students neither need nor want them. There is a paradox here. I have already referred to it, and I have tried to solve it by avoiding (almost!) all the maths and equations in the literature, merely (in the text) attributing the more entertaining remarks or observations to those who made them (e.g. on p. 49, 'as John Clarke has remarked in his tutorial series..') and at the end of the book telling where you can find out more if you wish.

Finally, a number of expressions of gratitude and acknowledgements of help are most certainly due. To those first of all who brought me up: my father, a general practitioner of 35 years standing, who taught me what medicine is about; my university teachers such as Professor Sir William Hodge, who taught me to think scientifically; and to surgeons such as Mr. Blacow Yates and Mr. Jimmy Lytle, who taught me to think surgically. To those friends and colleagues whose wisdom (not mine) fills this book – far too many to mention individually and most of them would be embarrassed to be singled out. To the students, for helpful, constructive, albeit sometimes critical, comments, and to those involved in the production of this small book, go my warmest appreciation.

F.T. de Dombal
Leeds, 1993

1

Introduction to surgical decision making

'Diagnosis', remarked a computing friend of mine to an astonished professor of surgery some time in the 1960s, 'is nothing more than classifying rocks or flowers or trees'. As you may imagine, it did not take the professor more than a few minutes to send him packing, which was a pity because he had a good deal to offer, and because in a sense both of them were right. What the computing expert was trying to say, perhaps imperfectly, was a point that has been made many times since – namely that diagnosis or decision making by intuition, guess or 'hunch' is difficult to defend in this day and age. What the professor of surgery was trying to express, again perhaps imperfectly, was that surgical diagnosis and decision making is quite different from the 'mere' classification procedures that are utilized in other more exact scientific disciplines.

Surgical decisions are often far from clear-cut. They are often taken under conditions of great uncertainty, and it therefore could be argued that the surgeon has more in common with a military commander, who has to send his troops into battle, knowing some will be killed, and trying to minimize this figure, than with a botanist or zoologist who classifies flowers, rocks or trees on a totally objective basis.

This lack of 'exactness' in surgical decision making is not a criticism, more a recognition of just how difficult surgical decision making is in the real world. Indeed, it is impossible to study surgeons and their decisions for any length of time without gaining enormous respect for those who, day in and day out, are forced to take life and death decisions on, sometimes, the flimsiest of evidence.

In the dim and distant past, I once expended a considerable amount of time and energy leafing through all the textbooks I could find in an attempt to discover the particular characteristics that marked out surgery and surgeons from the other remaining clinicians. Anyone wishing to repeat the exercise may do so, although it was in many ways a fruitless task. Apart from the obvious difference that surgeons tend to operate on patients whereas other clinicians do not (and even this difference is becoming eroded with the growth of invasive radiological and endoscopic interventional techniques), there seemed little to distinguish surgery or surgeons from the remainder of their clinical colleagues.

The search was not completely wasted, however, for one aspect emerged – an aspect of particular importance to surgeons and the practice of surgery, and this concerned *surgical decision making*. Unlike other clinical medical disciplines, decisions taken in surgery have about them an urgency and a finality that marks them out from other clinical decisions. It is, for example, possible to prescribe a trial dose of a drug and observe the response, discontinuing the drug if no value is obtained. It is even possible to reverse the effects of many drugs by prescribing an antagonist if the drug therapy originally prescribed seems to be doing harm. It is, however, often impossible to reverse the results of an operation once the decision to proceed with surgery has been made; this lends to surgical decision making a particular importance, which may go some way towards explaining the public image of the surgeon as a decisive, assertive individual.

In a way it could be argued that this merely means that surgeons are true inheritors of the traditional practice of medicine, which depends in turn upon the derivation of the word 'medicine'. Most people believe that the practice of medicine began with Hippocrates, but this is not so. The word medicine derives from the word *medix* – an Etruscan word (antedating both Greek and Roman civilizations), a word that has nothing whatsoever to do with clinical healthcare at all. In Etruscan days, a *medix* was not a doctor but a local magistrate usually in a small village, an individual whose function was to listen to the local problems in the village, and adjudicate upon them. Thus, in short, a *medix* was someone who listened to peoples' problems and made decisions which solved these problems for the members of the local population.

From Etruscan times to the beginning of the twentieth century, relatively little changed as regards clinical medicine and especially surgery. The number of operations technically possible (at least until the development of modern anaesthesia) was finite and relatively small, and communities of surgeons tended to be similarly small and select. As regards decision making, the young surgeon took part in a long 'apprentice-like' scheme, being attached to a surgical firm in which the young surgeon could work with and learn from a senior colleague at first hand.

Surgical decision making in the formal sense was little taught, and in truth little needed. The decisions made by a young surgeon tended to be those of his teacher (even in the first half of the twentieth century), because accumulated surgical wisdom, at least as regards general surgery or a major speciality such as orthopaedics, could be retained in the mind of a single individual. There was little need, or impetus, to question the precepts that were taught; and when a new operation became available (e.g. partial gastrectomy) or a new line of therapy emerged (e.g. appendicectomy for appendicitis rather than expectant treatment for 'typhlitis'), the young surgeon of those days tended merely to visit an experienced surgeon, learn the new technique at first hand, and return and apply it in his practice.

Therefore, surgical decision making, although never easy, was until recently relatively clear-cut, as was the process by which it was taught and learnt. In the last few decades, however, much has occurred to change this relatively comfortable situation, and the reasons for this are several. First, the scope of surgery has increased enormously, as we shall discuss later. Second, societal pressures have increased upon the surgeon. Along with the vastly increased potential for investigation and treatment, has come the realization that society simply cannot pay for everyone to have access to all of this; hence a need has emerged to impose what are known as cost constraints upon the delivery of health-care.

These two developments would in themselves pose a dilemma for the surgeon. Unfortunately however, they have occurred at a time when the need for health care and surgery is increasing (partly because of the increasing age of the general population) and at a time when public awareness, public expectations, and public debate about the value of medical treatments have all also increased. For this no doubt we can blame the media in part. It is only natural that if the public are made aware almost daily via television and/or radio programmes of high technology (and high cost) health-care, they would want the same standard of treatment for themselves should they fall ill. And as if all this was not enough, political and medico-legal considerations increase yet further the pressure on the surgical decision maker.

It is, therefore, difficult not to feel some sympathy for the young surgeon, caught up in these various dilemmas in the process of trying to arrive at a decision. But worse is to follow! We have not yet arrived at the root cause of the young surgeon's problems, which stems from the complexity of modern medicine and modern surgery (together with the educational dilemmas that this complexity imposes). If we consider just a few basic facts, the nature of the dilemma becomes apparent.

- First, the time available to 'learn' surgery is relatively finite.
- Second, the faculty available to teach young surgeons is relatively static. Indeed in the UK during the 1980s the total medical faculty declined by 9.6%.
- Finally, the amount to be learned by the aspiring surgeon, who wishes to bring up to date and optimal care to patients, has exploded.

Consider just these three facts for a moment, and it should not surprise you that current performance by junior surgeons fails to reach optimal or even satisfactory levels. It is not surprising that the diagnostic accuracy of the first doctor to see patients with acute abdominal pain in UK hospitals averages 45%. It is not surprising that around 30% of trauma deaths in the UK are deemed to be avoidable by an expert panel. It is not surprising that the 'lead time' between presentation to a clinician and diagnosis of gastro-intestinal cancer averages up to 48 weeks (depending on the site of the cancer). None of these things are surprising, because whilst clinical audit demonstrates that they exist, clinical information science demonstrates that they are *inevitable*.

This last point needs to be stressed again and again. Some of us realized what was happening over 20 years ago, and were much reviled at the time for drawing attention to the poor performance levels in various respects. We were accused of 'talking the profession down'. Twenty years later it is easy to understand both points of view. On the one hand we all tend somewhat to share the view of the fictional Dr. Pangloss – 'everything is for the best in the best of all possible worlds' – and it is always upsetting to have this 'presumption of regularity' challenged and overturned. On the other hand, the problems have not gone away. Indeed they have become worse over the last 20 years. The need for the undergraduate student and postgraduate surgeon to spend less time acquiring factual knowledge and more time thinking about decision making has become more and more pressing. Consider two further points.

- the factual basis supporting clinical medicine (the knowledge base) has been estimated at 15 000 000 facts, and is increasing rapidly
- on a good day, a good student can learn (and retain) about nine facts an hour.

Many medical schools and regulatory bodies now recognize the need for the inclusion of some form of instruction concerning decision making to be built into the undergraduate and postgraduate curricula. The Association of American Medical Colleges positively recommends it. But what is to be taught? What is surgical decision making? How is the decision making process structured? How can inexperienced surgeons best learn to take optimal decisions? We will deal with these fundamental matters in the remaining chapters, and of these perhaps the most basic of all is the nature of the decision making process itself. It is therefore with this process that we shall be concerned in the remaining pages of this chapter.

The decision making process

How do surgeons decide what to do with a particular patient? Until about 1960 (for reasons already specified) the simple answer is nobody knew – and nobody minded very much. During the 1960s however, there was a surge of interest in clinical decision making, and a number of studies were performed, which began for the first time to 'model' the decision making process of surgeons and, indeed, other doctors as well. Many of these studies were performed by decision analysts or psychological experts and the outcome was described in terms often incomprehensible to surgeons, the present author amongst them! Nevertheless from these various studies a consensus view began to emerge of the steps involved in the medical decision making process and the consensus view is outlined in Figure 1.1. From this figure it will be seen that there are essentially three steps in the process.

- First, the surgeon needs to *acquire information from the patient*, because without adequate and appropriate information, no sensible decision can be taken.
- Second, the *information needs to be analysed* in order to assess the situation. Notice here that there is a difference between 'analysis of the information' and 'arriving at a diagnosis'. This distinction is deliberate. As later chapters will demonstrate, there is far more to the decision making process than simply making a diagnosis (in the sense of 'tying a label to each patient'), and as before the analysis of patient information needs to be appropriate and adequate if a sensible decision is to be made.
- Finally, following appropriate acquisition of information and equally appropriate analysis, a *decision about management* is made. Once again, there is more to the decision making process than simply 'deciding what to do'. The surgeon needs to know the range of options available in the particular circumstances, and the patient's wishes – and additionally, the likelihood of success and the consequences both of success and of failure. Addi-

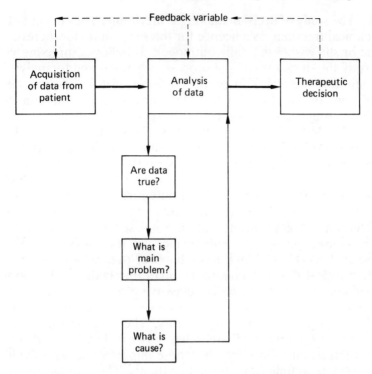

Figure 1.1 Illustration of the main elements of the surgical decision making process, representing consensus view of the 1960s and 1970s studies by a variety of authors. (From de Dombal F T (1979) Computers and the surgeon: a matter of decision. Nyhus L M, ed. *Surgery Annual*, 32–57.)

tionally, ethical conflicts (where these occur) need to be reviewed.

These then are the main elements of the decision making process: (i) information acquisition; (ii) information analysis; and (iii) management decision. They are actually the main steps in making *any* decision; but as you may already suspect, surgery imposes some special conditions upon each step. Each will be considered in turn in the next chapters. For now however, some brief concluding remarks are appropriate to summarize the main points of the present broad introduction to the subject.

1. The study of decision making is inevitable. The concept of 'clinical freedom' as a licence for the surgeon to do whatever he or she wishes is totally outmoded. It behoves surgeons to study the decision making process in general and to analyse their own decisions in particular – mostly for the pressing reasons outlined earlier but also because every surgeon is increasingly called upon to justify (publicly) actions taken.

2. The decision making process is sequential. It is wildly optimistic (and very foolish) to assume that mistakes made at an earlier stage of the process can be rectified later on. For example, failure to acquire adequate and appropriate information from a patient can only rarely be remedied by even the most complex of analyses or the most inspired of decisions. If appropriate data are not secured, or the analysis is not appropriate, only by luck will the correct decision be arrived at – and luck has a habit of running out!

3. Surgical decision making involves uncertainty. Decision making in surgery is *not* like classifying rocks or flowers. It involves making important decisions sometimes under conditions of considerable uncertainty. The surgeon therefore needs to understand firstly, that surgical decisions will be imperfect, and secondly, that these imperfect decisions will from time to time cause harm to patients. The surgeon needs to come to terms with this; and it is better to do so by an understanding of what the decision making process is about than by hiding behind a cloak of 'clinical freedom', or (worse) 'my experience'.

4. Decision making is (in principle) quite simple. Decision making can be made very difficult, particularly when 'formal' (usually meaning mathematical) decision making is discussed. Indeed, the way some 'experts' in the field carry on, one might imagine they had a vested interest in making things difficult! The prudent surgeon is interested in such concepts, but not slavishly bound by them – and in day to day work practices (rather than rigorous mathematical decision making) what is known as 'Objective Medical Decision Making' (OMDM).

OMDM seeks to ensure that all surgical decisions are made on the basis of accurately collected, appropriate and adequate evidence, following thorough review and appropriate analysis in the mind of the surgeon. OMDM should be (and is) welcome to most surgeons, because it represents a return to the traditional values of clinical medicine, with its emphasis particularly upon history taking and physical examination and the need to talk to patients carefully and to examine meticulously.

As such, although the surgeon might well be wary of (difficult to understand) mathematical analyses and flow diagrams, which sometimes seem to have little to do with clinical reality, it is scarcely possible to argue with the central premise of OMDM, 'do it right, get it right!' We shall explore how to do it right and therefore get it right in the next few chapters.

2

Obtaining, recording and transmitting good information

In Chapter 1 we considered some of the basic steps in the decision making process, and you will recall that the first of these basic steps concerned obtaining adequate and appropriate information from the patient.

This step is by far the most important, because if this part of the process is carried out badly, or inadequately, then all is lost. It should scarcely be necessary to make this point, but unfortunately it is. There seems to be a distressing tendency to believe, particularly, for some reason, in North America, that high technology can overcome deficiencies in interview and examination technique.

Of course it cannot, but doctors are not alone in thinking that it can. Many of my computing friends spend their days writing ever more complex programs based around ever more intricate techniques of 'artificial intelligence' designed to remedy poor interview and examination technique. 'Neural networks' are in current vogue: by the time you read this, 'chaos theory' may have taken over. This application of high technology or artificial intelligence is mere wishful thinking. No amount of convoluted thinking on your part will remedy the situation if you regularly make mistakes during the interview or examination, and/or order too many investigations, the wrong investigations, or as it sometimes seems random investigations in an attempt to solve the problem you yourself have created.

No doctor has the right to talk about a difficult case (or talk about a difficult decision) unless information has been sought from the patient in a thorough, relevant, accurate, and comprehensible fashion. So in this chapter we are going to look at the process of obtaining, recording and transmitting good information from the patient ('good' in the sense we have just defined). Now of course it is impossible in a single chapter to deal with each specific symptom or physical sign; so what I propose to do in the next few pages is to concentrate on some general principles involved in interviewing, examining and investigating patients (and in recording and transmitting the information you gather), to deal with some of the common pitfalls in a way that may help you improve your own technique, and in particular to discuss with you the *purpose* of each of these aspects – on the basis that if you do not know *why* you are doing something, you are unlikely to do it to the best of your ability.

The patient interview

Careful studies by senior physicians have shown that in over 80% of patients in whom a correct diagnosis is eventually made, the correct diagnosis is already suspected by the physician after the clinical interview, before any physical findings have been elicited and before any investigations have been performed. In clinical surgery the picture may be a little different because some patients present with superficial lesions, and here the diagnosis is mostly visual. However, the same broad principle applies. Improving one's interview technique is the single most important step that can be taken along the road to better diagnosis and better decision making.

Unfortunately, one has only to watch a number of clinical interviews carried out by sensible medical students or inexperienced surgeons, to realize that literally as well as figuratively the people concerned do not know what they are doing. That is to say there is no sense of purpose behind the interview. Questions are being asked by rote, sometimes it seems at random, rather than with a specific purpose in mind. It may therefore be helpful, before saying a few words about interview technique, to discuss why we interview the patient in the first place.

The how and why of clinical interviews

Any moderately extensive surgical textbook will inform you *how* to conduct a clinical interview. Indeed, most medical students in their first day or two on the wards are instructed to interview the patient along the following lines:

- introduction to the patient
- list of presenting complaint(s)
- history of the presenting complaint(s)
- their associated symptoms
- systematic inquiry
- past and social medical history.

Unfortunately, students are not taught *why* they are going through this procedure, and the reasons both for the procedure and for teaching it to students are quite complex. After a little while, many medical students become quite confused concerning clinical interviewing. 'They teach one thing and do another' is a familiar complaint.

I have some sympathy with this problem but not a lot, because it indicates principally that the medical student or young surgeon has never really stopped to consider why he or she is being taught to take a history in this comprehensive fashion. It needs to be reiterated that the aim of the clinical interview, as carried out when the patient is first seen in the Emergency Room or the surgery wards, is not merely to make a diagnosis. The aims are in fact much more complex, along the following lines:

- to establish a rapport with the patient
- to identify the patient's main problem or problems
- to get some idea of the cause of the problems
- to identify other problems (medical and/or social) related to the disease or its management
- to build patient confidence.

The first and most important of these is establishment of rapport with the patient. This comes easily to some, but if you are not a fortunate 'natural communicator' this aspect above all else is the one that you should concentrate upon during your training. Other skills can be picked up from textbooks or check-lists but the establishment of rapport with the patient can only be acquired (unless it comes naturally) from continual practise or considerable experience.

Sometimes, it is only after establishing a rapport with the patient that you can understand and identify the patient's problem. Remember in this context that you cannot solve the problem until you have defined it. Defining the problem may be amongst the more difficult tasks of the clinical interview, because it may not be the obvious problem of which the patient complains, but it is this ability that marks out the doctor or surgeon from others (such as paramedics) who may be superb at following check-lists but less so at solving problems for patients.

Interview technique

The technique of clinical interview has been the subject of several excellent textbooks and it is only possible here to offer some general guidelines, which may help you to avoid the common pitfalls. In outline, to carry out an effective clinical interview, you need a number of skills, for example:

- you need to ask the right questions
- you need to ask the questions right
- you need to understand the answers.

Rule 1. Ask the right questions

First of all, what are the 'right questions'? This is where most medical students and junior surgeons go wrong. They imagine the right questions are simply those which lead to the correct diagnosis. Remember, however, we have just discussed the various purposes of the clinical interview; and we have agreed that there is far more to the interview than mere diagnosis. It is consideration of *all* these purposes which defines the 'right questions to ask'. It is consideration of these purposes which explains *why* students are taught to take a history in the fashion described. The 'right questions' in a given situation are those that achieve the purposes set out on p. 12. No more and no less.

Let us look forward in the book for a concrete example. As we shall discuss in Chapter 5, you have little hope of correctly diagnosing a patient with acute abdominal pain without asking the relevant questions in Figure 5.3 on p. 72. However, if you want to carry out a thorough interview there is more to it than that, because if your purpose is to identify problems, for example relating to management, you cannot hope simply to confine yourself to questions concerning diagnosis. You must ask other questions as well – questions about past problems, cardiovascular symptoms, and so on – *which do not affect diagnosis but may influence your management.*

Most students get confused here, and so do quite a number of young surgeons. There are over 1000 possible questions that *could* be asked, and because students or young surgeons do not know why they are asking the questions, they do not know which questions to choose. Often they fall back on conducting a 'systematic enquiry' and asking questions about past and social history, usually asking those questions they were taught in medical school, often without much relevance to the case in question.

You can solve this dilemma by looking at it from another angle. Once you have identified the patient's problem, what is the point of any further questioning? The history of the presenting complaint clearly needs to be analysed in detail, because this will help you identify the likely cause of the problem, and its extent and severity.

The point of almost all the remaining interview questions is quite different, namely to identify problems that might affect (or be affected by) the management of the patient. If you learn to think in this fashion, then the point of the exercise (and the questions to ask) both become much clearer. To give just two examples, if you are proposing to operate on a particular patient, timely questions such as whether the patient has diabetes or chronic obstructive airways disease, may help anticipate and prevent post-operative problems. Similarly in an elderly patient, questions concerning the social situation may help anticipate and prevent problems when the time comes for the patient to leave hospital.

Rule 2. Ask the questions right

So clearly you need to ask the right questions; but also asking the questions right is equally important. It never fails to amaze me how many students and inexperienced surgeons do not seem to consider this aspect. Perhaps they feel the questions are so obvious that they cannot cause confusion. Well, they might be obvious to the surgeon but they are not obvious to other people! During the 1970s we carried out studies in which three doctors stood behind a senior clinician and a patient, and noted down the conversation. Some 20% of the surgeon's questions were so vaguely phrased that three other clinicians could not even agree what questions were being asked, and 16% of the patient's answers were so vague the same three clinicians could not agree whether the patient had said yes or no.

Let us explore this vital point further. As an exercise in your own interview technique consider three aspects of pain: (i) the site at onset; (ii) aggravating factors; and (iii) the type of pain. Ask yourself, how would you enquire about these points? If you are being honest, it is probably along the following lines:

- Where was the pain when it came on?
- Does anything make the pain worse?
- What is the pain like?

These questions represent what most people ask. They sound reasonable. They are not. The first (concerning site of pain at onset) may elicit any answer from 'Tuesday' (the patient thought you said 'when did the pain come on?') to 'here' pointing to the site of pain at present (the patient thought you said 'where is the pain when it comes on?').

The second question usually elicits incomprehension – so you give the patient examples. 'Is it worse when you cough?' (yes doctor); 'Is it worse when you move?' (yes doctor); 'Is it worse when you stand on your head?' (yes doctor). Some patients will say yes to anything because they have not understood and they are trying to be polite. Even worse, the third question is often asked so vaguely as to be almost meaningless. You may well understand what you mean by 'boring', 'burning', 'stabbing' and so on and the patient may understand what he or she means by them, but unfortunately only rarely do these impressions coincide.

All of these pitfalls are avoidable. The first can be avoided by: (a) establishing where the pain is right now; (b) asking whether the pain was *ever* anywhere else, (c) asking when the pain *first* came on; and (d) asking where was the pain *at that time*. The second problem can be avoided by asking the patient to do something (e.g. to move or cough) while watching to see if it clearly hurts, and if it does, asking the patient to point to the site of pain. Finally, the third pitfall can be averted by characterizing the pain as steady, colicky or intermittent rather than using some vague term like burning or stabbing, making sure of course that *you* know what these terms mean and that you phrase the questions so that the patient can understand (e.g. 'is there ever a time when the pain goes away completely?' not, 'is your pain intermittent?').

Rule 3. Assess the answers correctly
The third and last point concerning interview technique is a simple one. If your interview technique is to be effective you need to assess the accuracy of the answers which the patient is giving you. Textbooks will point out that ideally questions should be all phrased so as to provide yes or no answers, and this is true, because observer variation studies have shown that this type of answer is reproducible, whereas answers giving 'opinions' are so open to variation between observers as to be almost meaningless.

There is, however, more to it than that. You need to assess carefully whether or not a patient has understood the question in the first place. You need to know the difference between information (what you think you said) and knowledge (what the patient thinks you said). You need to remember that patients are apprehensive, and tend to smile and nod even when they do not understand at all (or have misheard you).

So in summing up the clinical interview remember that, although potentially quite simple, it has many pitfalls. In particular remember *why* you are interviewing the patient in the first place; remember to ask the right questions; remember to ask them in the right way; and finally remember that the patient may have totally misunderstood (and you therefore may have totally misunderstood the patient's answer). If you can remember all of these things, and adapt your own interview technique accordingly, then you should be well on the way to conducting effective interviews.

Physical examination

Here we encounter some substantial difference between physicians and surgeons, because in surgery the physical examination has a special importance. My physician colleagues will deny this, pointing out that physicians are perfectly capable of exemplary examination of the patient. Nevertheless, as we have already seen, the physician has made a tentative correct diagnosis in 80% or 90% of the time after interview alone. Surgical diagnosis often contains a visual element, which is not found in internal medicine, such as in relation to minor superficial conditions (e.g. skin lesions). This is often called 'spot diagnosis', and is particularly beloved of examiners. As with the interview, so once again in relation to physical examination it is worth considering some principles and pitfalls to sharpen up your technique.

The aims of physical examination

The student or young surgeon who has not thought beyond the principles of 'spot diagnosis' to consider the *purpose* of physical examination, will fail to carry out this procedure appropriately and effectively. As with the interview, the purpose of physical examination is not just to decide the diagnosis, but is more complex than this. The ideal physical examination would do a number of things:

- confirm or refute hypotheses generated by the interview.
- provide evidence concerning the possible cause of the patient's problem.

- provide evidence concerning severity and extent of disease
- form a basis for decision concerning patient management
- do all of this without discomfort to the patient.

Technique of physical examination
Everything we discussed concerning the need for precision and attention to detail in relation to the clinical interview applies also to the physical examination. You cannot, for example, hope to diagnose a squamous cell carcinoma by its raised, rolled, everted edge unless you know a raised, rolled, everted edge when you see it. You cannot assess the value of Murphy's sign unless you know what Murphy's sign is. You cannot appreciate the significance of rebound tenderness unless you know exactly how to go about eliciting it. Some time ago at an extremely prestigeous North American medical school, I was disappointed, but not surprised, to find that eight different senior residents in the front row came up with five different definitions of rebound tenderness when asked precisely this question.

The guidance that can be offered in this small volume can in no way take the place of the many excellent textbooks already available. (For example, if you have not already read Hamilton Bailey's, *Physical Signs*, why not!) Nevertheless, there are some general rules to help you, using the skill and experience you possess, to improve the effectiveness of your own examination.

Rule 1. Define physical signs meticulously
It is fairly obvious that your examination technique will not be meticulous unless you understand very precisely the definitions of the physical signs you are looking for.

There are over 1 000 recognized physical signs (many eponymous) and a single example will have to suffice. Earlier, we discussed rebound tenderness. Before reading on, think about your own definition of rebound tenderness, and then compare your definition with the definition arrived at by a consensus of over 500 surgeons. In this definition, in order to elicit rebound tenderness there are three steps as follows:

- Press on the appropriate area sufficiently hard to depress the peritoneum. This is painful (otherwise rebound tenderness is not present).
- Wait for a few moments, sufficient for the peritoneum to accommodate itself to the new position. The pain decreases.
- Remove your hand smartly to skin level but not beyond. The peritoneum will 'bound back' to its original position and the patient will feel pain (often with a reflex inspiration).

If your own definition matches that set out above, then fine. If you elicit rebound tenderness in any other way you may make errors, particularly false positive errors, in your elicitation of rebound tenderness. If (like one of the residents discussed above) you imagine rebound tenderness involves pressing on the left side of the abdomen and thereby eliciting pain in the right lower quadrant (which is in fact Røvsing's sign) you are unlikely to get the maximum value from this test.

Rule 2. Remember the purposes of the examination
It helps, while examining a patient, to keep in mind *why* you are doing this. Remember that the prime purpose of physical examination is to confirm the initial hypothesis concerning the disease and its management, which you have formed as a result of the clinical interview. Recall also that your own ability to remember is limited. This is why most experienced examiners examine the relevant area (the abdomen or whatever) while the features of the clinical interview are still fresh in their mind.

While conducting your examination it also helps to keep in mind that you are not merely doing so in order to make a diagnosis but in order to form a basis for patient management. There are two good reasons why diagnosis is not enough and more information is needed. First, severity and extent of disease may be more important in terms of patient management than the mere presence or absence of a particular diagnosis (e.g. severity of inflammatory bowel disease, or extent of spread of carcinoma). Second, your decision concerning management may be influenced by other conditions quite apart from the patient's main problem. (For example, early breast cancer in a fit 70-year-old woman would probably be managed differently from extensive breast cancer in a frail 80 year old who has already had two myocardial infarctions and a stroke.) So when faced with statements in the textbooks and on the wards concerning 'the need to examine the whole patient' remember the point of doing so is to enable you to make management decisions.

Rule 3. Remember the patient's feelings
Obviously it is not your intention in examining the patient to hurt or embarrass them. However, both may be inevitable, and there is an important point to remember here. If you have a physical sign to elicit which you feel will hurt or embarrass the patient leave it until the last. We discussed rebound tenderness earlier. Properly elicited, this is painful. You will get no more cooperation from a patient after this! So in examining the abdomen, for example, I recommend you adopt a slightly different sequence from that in most textbooks – first observing the abdomen, then listening to it, then percussing it, then feeling lightly for tenderness and only then proceeding to attempt to elicit rebound tenderness. (This may still hurt but then at least you can reassure the patient that the examination is over.) You will often find that your chief instinctively follows this sequence – leaving embarrassing or painful physical signs right until the end of the physical examination. It is a very good plan to adopt, and I suggest you do so at an early stage of your career.

Guidelines for investigation of patients

I do not know the total number of investigations available to the surgeon. And if I did know, I would not tell you – for two reasons. First, because by the time you read the book the information would be out of date. Second, in investigating a patient you should not be thinking of the maximum number of investigations you can perform, but of the *minimum* number of investigations necessary to resolve a patient's particular problem.

If you really want to read a dissertation on the finer points of a raised serum vanadium level (or whatever), by all means look elsewhere. But in doing so, beware! Remember that the more information you have the less likely you will be able to analyse it. This particularly applies to biochemical data, where test results tend to come in batches of a dozen figures at a time and where previous studies have shown that surgeons obtain masses of relatively useless data – in that they utilize less than 5% of it, and then do not utilize it in a sensible or appropriate way. Some time ago the *Lancet* (acidly, but in my view realistically) referred editorially to this process as 'biochemical bingo'.

So by all means, if you wish, consult an appropriate textbook for detailed information about the serum vanadium or the faecal neptunium, because you will not find it here. Here we are concerned not with performing every possible test but performing just enough tests to enable us to manage the patient, and no more.

The aims of investigation

As with clinical interview and physical examination, investigation of the patient is performed for a specific purpose, or at least it should be. All too often the student or young surgeon has little idea *why* an investigation is being performed. All too often an investigation is performed 'because that is what is done here'. This is quite wrong. Any investigation should not be ordered unless it is likely to accomplish one of the following purposes:

• steer the clinician towards a correct diagnosis
• decrease the likelihood of a possible alternative diagnosis
• establish the severity and/or extent of disease
• uncover (or rule out) other problems likely to affect management

- increase certainty so that a management decision can be made.

If none of these purposes can be accomplished, the test should not be done. I suggest therefore, that in deciding which or how many investigations are appropriate for a particular patient at a particular time in their illness, you would do well to remember that every item of additional information tends to confuse as well as possibly help. The overriding principle of your investigational strategy should not be how many tests you can perform but how few tests you can perform (providing of course that the tests you perform lead you to the appropriate management). In doing so, there are a few guidelines to keep in mind, which will help you perform the minimum of tests with the maximum of effectiveness.

Rule 1. Beware (thoughtless) 'routine' investigations
No investigation should be performed until appropriate and adequate clinical interview and physical examination have been carried out. You may have noticed an increasing tendency to perform what are labelled 'basic tests' on every patient who walks through the door. I personally believe this is wrong. Only after you have thoroughly interviewed and examined a patient, and assessed the data appropriately, should you make up a list of investigations – and then the shortest possible list.

Rule 2. Know what you want from the test
Remember what has been said time and time again in this chapter. There is more to patient management than merely 'making the diagnosis'. When you are deciding which tests to order, remember that the management of the patient will involve: (a) making a diagnosis; (b) assessing the severity and extent of disease; and (c) making a management decision. Before you write out a lengthy list of investigational requests, ask yourself – which investigations are necessary to establish the correct diagnosis? Which investigations are necessary to establish the severity and extent of disease?

Which investigations are necessary to make an appropriate management decision for this patient?

These considerations should determine your list of requested investigations, and of course, the opposite is also true. An investigation should not appear on your list of requests unless it is likely to help you in making a diagnosis, assessing the severity and extent of disease, and above all making a management decision. If you cannot thoroughly justify an investigation under one of these headings, you should not be doing the investigation at all.

Rule 3. Know the test concerned
One of the reasons why special investigations are so ineffectively used is that those ordering the investigations do not know what to make of the results. In the world of computers and diagnosis, you may have seen articles which argue very strongly that computer aided diagnosis is dangerous if the doctor in question does not know the computer's track record. Even as a computer buff, I personally agree with this, but it clearly also extends to every other investigation. An investigation should not be performed unless someone familiar with the test, the result patterns, their implications, and the limitations of the investigation is going to look at the data. If you do not know what to make of the results you should not be ordering the investigation in the first place.

Rule 4. Minimize invasiveness
We shall talk in the next chapter about the value of tests and how they may contribute to reducing uncertainty. For now, remember that if two tests have a similar value in a particular situation, the test you should choose is that which is going to cause the patient less upset. Such a policy seems blindingly obvious, but as we shall see this is merely a special case of a more general problem.

Rule 5. Do not delay the decision
All tests have a cost. Some cost the patient discomfort and some cost the health care delivery system money. You know this perfectly well. There is, however, a further hidden cost,

which applies to every investigation, and that is the cost in time. An investigation should not delay a management decision unnecessarily, and above all an investigation should not substitute for management decision. The test I like to see least of all is the innocuous but useless test ordered 5 min before the young surgeon is due to go off duty. It tells me little about the patient, but tells me a great deal about the young surgeon who uses such a device to duck the necessity of decision making.

Recording and transmitting information

Getting good information from the patient is all very well, but it is often not much use if you keep it to yourself. So in the final section of this chapter we need to look at some of the problems in recording and transmitting information to other people, and in particular we need to look at the problems that surround the 'case record'.

This is another bone of contention between students and their teachers. Most students are asked to write 'case notes' about the patients they see. They expend considerable time and effort in doing this (often without knowing *why* they are doing it), and they get more than a little depressed when they and their deathless prose encounter one of two serious problems.

First, students are taught to write out a 'full case history' – and then find they cannot do this in real life after they qualify, because there simply is no time. This leads, after qualification amongst other things, to poor handwriting, illegible case notes, and personalized abbreviations (e.g. PERLA, L/R, =, which indicates that the pupils are equal in size and react to light and accommodation, I think).

Second, the student writes out a case history and presents to a Dr. X. This is immediately criticized and the student is told to redo it in a different (often idiosyncratic) fashion. The student then moves to a different firm, only to be shouted at by a Dr. Y, who insists upon case histories written in what appears to be a completely different fashion. After a few firms the student loses heart and eventually does what he or she is told in a disgruntled fashion.

The reason this situation comes about is because the student has never considered (and never even been encouraged to consider) what the *aims* of the case record are, and what the *criteria* are by which case records should be judged. The aims of the case record include the following:

- documentation of the patient's problem to allow appropriate management decisions
- documentation to form a baseline for future change in the patient's condition
- basis for communication to others involved in the patient's health-care
- basis for medico-legal evidence if appropriate
- basis for research and teaching.

So, to the question 'are your case-notes appropriate', the answer is simple. If your case notes allow the preceding aims to be fulfilled then they are adequate. If they do not allow the above aims to be fulfilled, they are inadequate. Any further 'fine tuning' of the case notes represents merely the style of Dr. X (or Dr. Y) and is of secondary consideration. What you should therefore do after writing out your own case notes for a particular patient is to ask yourself – do my case notes allow the above aims to be fulfilled? If they do, they are adequate. If they do not, they are inadequate and you need to change them. It is as simple as that.

As regards documentation of the patient's problem (and acting as a baseline), we have already discussed many of the items that need to go in your case records. As regards communicating information to others, the question you need to ask yourself is also simple. Imagine that your case notes have been written by somebody else, and you are reviewing the patient having just returned from holiday. Could you (quickly, easily and accurately) inform yourself of the patient's problem? Could you make appropriate management decisions on the basis of what is in the case notes? If you could, your case notes are adequate and Dr. X (or Dr. Y) is just being idiosyncratic. If you could not, your case notes are inadequate.

There is another aspect of communication that puzzles most students. When they are asked to 'present a case' at the chief's grand round, they are required to do so in a long-winded and laborious way, going over every one of the items of information they have gathered. Woe betide the student who fails to mention that the patient once had a (totally irrelevant) operation to remove an ingrowing toenail 20 years ago! Students are somewhat puzzled when it appears that amongst senior surgical staff, cases are discussed in a totally different manner. Again I sympathize, but not much. Such students have failed to realize that the purpose of students presenting a case in this long-winded fashion is to enable their teachers to be assured that the student has asked all the possible questions correctly and has got the appropriate answers. It has nothing at all to do with effective communication in real life.

In order to practise effective communication of your information to others, write out a 'short' case history on half a sheet of paper. Now, imagine you are a surgical registrar and your house surgeon rings you at 3 a.m. (when you are asleep) about a new patient. Go through your 'short' case history. Can you understand clearly, in a few sentences, what the patient's problem is and make a management decision on this basis? If you can, the communication is effective. If you cannot, it is not.

Finally, if you want to practise effective communication, there is a quick, easy (and fun) way. Enlist the help of a medical student friend; give the friend your case notes about a patient you have seen. *After 2 or 3 min only* ask your friend what the patient's problem is (and what he or she is going to do about it). If your friend can work this out easily from your case notes, they are adequate, and if not, they are inadequate. (Similarly try picking up an imaginary telephone and talking to your friend for 90 seconds, no more, and see what your friend makes of the situation.) This is excellent practice. It is also sometimes great fun, and if you learn to behave in this fashion you will at least have the satisfaction of knowing that in obtaining and communicating information you are behaving like a surgeon and not like a clerk.

3
Weighing up the evidence

After interviewing a patient, performing physical examination, and with the results of appropriate special investigations to hand, the next step in the decision making process is to weigh up the evidence.

In practice, as you will see by referring back to Figure 1.1 on p. 7, the process is an 'iterative' one. The result of a special investigation may lead you to a new train of thought which necessitates going back to the patient and asking some further questions or clarifying specific points. Thus, finding glucose in the urine on routine testing may alert you to the need to go back to the patient, question the patient closely about possible diabetes, and look again for the stigmata of this condition, which may have escaped your notice on the first occasion. We will for now, however, assume the information you have got is complete and the next step is to analyse this information.

As before, you need to be clear in your own mind as to exactly *why* you are analysing the information. Most students, when this question is posed, respond that they are trying to make a diagnosis. So it needs to be emphasized once again here that the purpose of analysing the information is ultimately to make a decision about the patient, and hence there is more than one question to be answered:

- is the information true?
- what is the patient's problem?
- what is the most likely disease category?
- what other diseases need to be considered?
- how severe is the disease?
- Are any other conditions likely to affect management?

Remember the ultimate goal of analysing patient information is to make an appropriate decision. All of the considerations on this list should be going through your mind when
you weigh up the evidence from the patient. We shall look at
some ways of doing this, but first there are a couple more
considerations that need to be discussed – namely (i) the
limitations of the human mind and (ii) the differences
between what are known as determinist and probabilist
approaches.

Limitations of the human mind

Here we come face to face with a problem that troubles
many students when they first enter clinical medicine. You
are taught to take a 'full' case history and are frequently
chastised when you fail to repeat some of this information at
the chief's next round. You then watch the chief ignoring all
of these principles, asking half a dozen questions, and
making an accurate diagnosis! This puzzles many students,
and it distresses some, but it need not do so if they realize
what is going on. Remember, students are not taught to take
a full case history because all of the facts are relevant in
every case, but because their teachers need to know that
they have acquired the necessary skills to elicit all of this
information thoroughly and accurately (see p. 24).

It is important to realize that information is *not* all of
equal value when it comes to weighing up the evidence and
deciding what to do with the patient. This is somewhat
fortunate, because numerous studies have shown that the
human mind has very severe limitations when it comes to
weighing up evidence. If you want the jargon terminology,
the human mind functions like an information system of
limited channel capacity. Put more simply, this means we
can generally remember and evaluate only about seven
things at once (some people a few more, some a few less). In
case you are wondering, studies have shown that doctors are
no different from the rest of the population in this regard
(Figure 3.1).

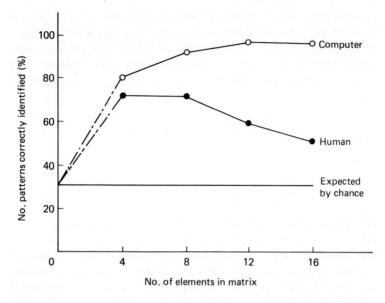

Figure 3.1 Influence of amount of information on diagnostic accuracy for (a) humans and (b) computers. Note that the computer accuracy increases with more information, whereas human accuracy falls with increasing information. (From de Dombal F T, Horrocks J C, Staniland J R *et al.* (1992) *Methods of Information in Medicine*; **11**: 32–7.)

Heuristic behaviour

The implications of this are extremely important. What it means is that although you may well have been encouraged to take a full case history, you have no hope whatsoever of analysing each item of information in it. Experienced surgeons have learned this the hard way. The experienced surgeon, given a clue that suggests a particular disease, (e.g. acute appendicitis), will immediately focus down on the half a dozen or so items, which (by experience) he or she has learnt most likely to confirm or refute this diagnosis. This type of behaviour is known as 'heuristic' and is a particular characteristic of the way that senior surgeons as opposed to inexperienced surgeons approach a diagnostic problem.

This concept of 'heuristic' behaviour allows you to understand what your chief is doing. Your chief has learned (from years of experience) 'short lists' of valuable symptoms and signs relating to each clinical situation and (instinctively recognizing the limitations of the human mind) is exhibiting what the psychologists call 'goal-seeking' or 'heuristic' behaviour. If the chief's 'pet' questions produce the required answer the chief will look no further. If on the other hand they do not, then the chief will switch to an alternative line of questioning.

Computer aided studies show this rather well. Look at a real life example (Figure 3.2 and 3.3). Both figures concern the same patient and they illustrate, question by question, the probabilities of various common diseases after each question put to the patient. The first figure, Figure 3.2, illustrates the approach of a senior registrar, and the probabilities shown are those for the common causes of acute abdominal pain (which was the reason for the patient's admission to hospital). As you can see, after a few questions the senior registrar obtains a clue that the patient may have a particular disease (acute appendicitis) and in the figure you can see clearly how the senior registrar cashes in on this clue by following up with several key questions designed to establish beyond doubt in his own mind the diagnosis of acute appendicitis (which was correct in this instance).

This is an example of 'heuristic' or 'goal seeking' behaviour. In this type of behaviour, the subject behaves like a rat in an experimental maze, trying one avenue of approach after another, then following the right one to the goal. Figure 3.2 is an ideal example and you may think it is so simple that everyone automatically follows this pathway. Not so: in Figure 3.3 we can see the way the house surgeon tackled the same case. In practice, the house surgeon got the same clue, but failed to appreciate its significance, and after eleven or twelve questions (chosen, it seems, almost at random), the probabilities of diseases are all about the same. It is not difficult to see why in this instance the house surgeon made the wrong diagnosis and called the registrar, with the results we have already seen.

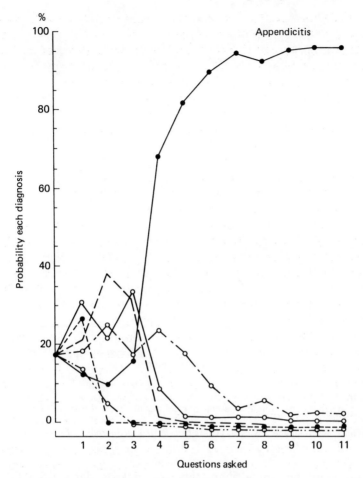

Figure 3.2. Analysis of heuristic behaviour shown by a senior registrar dealing with a patient suffering from acute abdominal pain. Linear figure indicates probability of common diseases after each question. Note how, when one 'clue' is obtained, the senior registrar pursues hypothesis and confirms it, correctly. This is heuristic behaviour. (From Leaper D J, Gill P W, Staniland J R *et al.* (1973) *British Medical Journal*; 569–74.

Next time you stand behind the chief, watch out for this 'heuristic' type of questioning. (No, I did not mean to imply your chief was a rat, or behaved like one, but merely that

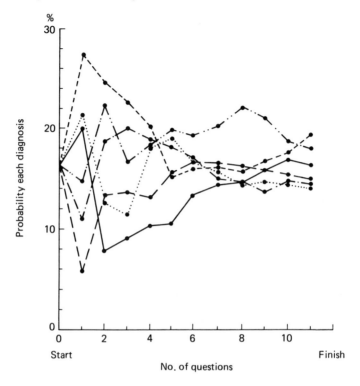

Figure 3.3 Same patient as in Figure 3.2, but showing the analysis of a house surgeon's questions. Note that although 'clue' was obtained, it was not pursued. This is not heuristic behaviour, and is manifestly not effective. (From Leaper D J, Gill P W, Staniland J R *et al.* (1973) *British Medical Journal*; : 569–74.)

your chief has an efficient way of making decisions.) Of course you would like to do this yourself and probably in the fullness of time you will come to behave in this way as well; but for now you face a problem in that you are not sure what are the 'best questions to ask'. Later in this book we will discuss one or two specific clinical situations, and provide you with some lists to start you off. For now the important points to remember are:

- not all information is of equal weight
- you can only take in half a dozen or so facts at once

- you therefore need to distinguish (for each clinical situation) between information that is critical and useful, and that which is merely interesting.

Determinist and probabilist approaches

In weighing up the evidence you will also come up against another important problem that relates particularly to clinical medicine. This concerns the difference between 'determinist' and 'probabilist' information. To understand the differences between these two types of information, think back to Chapter 1, my former computing friend and his rocks, flowers and trees.

If one is trying to identify a type of tree, the way in which one does this is by a 'determinist' approach. The leaves are of such and such shape, the bark of the tree is such and such texture, the colour is such and such, and so on. At the end of this process, the tree is identified. There is virtually never any doubt. The leaves are of the particular shape, or they are not. The tree is evergreen, or it is deciduous. It is either an oak tree or it is not. These decisions are made on *determinist* information (features are either present or absent, and where present, then they are present in every tree).

The problem is that clinical medicine is not like that. First, the features themselves may be difficult to elicit, and although you may do your best to elicit rebound tenderness accurately and meticulously, even in the best hands the presence or absence of rebound tenderness may be in doubt in a small percentage of cases. (In less skilled hands, the doubt may extend to quite a large percentage.) Worse, in clinical medicine, not all features of a disease are present all the time. Palm trees do not grow acorns. Oak trees never grow coconuts. So if you see a tree bearing acorns or coconuts you immediately know what sort of tree you are dealing with. However, not all patients with acute appendicitis have typical right lower quadrant pain and tenderness. In contrast some patients who do *not* have acute appendicitis may yet present with these typical features.

Weighing up clinical evidence

This is what makes the weighing up of evidence in clinical medicine so difficult, and is why some people describe the process as *probabilist*. Only rarely is a single appearance absolutely pathognomonic (specific for a particular disease, such as the typical rash of measles or smallpox). This leads to a number of problems and these can be best summarized as follows:

- most diagnoses are made on the basis of a *combination* of symptoms and signs, which (taken together) favour a particular disease category
- only rarely will *all* these 'typical' symptoms and signs be present in an individual case
- only rarely therefore, will a diagnosis be absolutely certain. Most often it will be *probable* rather than certain.

To illustrate this point let us compare determinist and probabilist approaches. In doing so, you will see that the determinist approach is certainly more simple (and is the approach followed in most textbooks). You will also see that the probabilist approach (although more complex) is capable of providing much more rich information about the patient and the disease. Consider the histopathological diagnosis of Crohn's disease and consider two 'typical' features, namely *granulomata* and *giant cells*. The determinist approach leads to statements such as the following:

giant cells and/or granulomata are said to be

- 'present in Crohn's disease'
- 'indicative of Crohn's disease'
- 'diagnostic for Crohn's disease'.

All of these statements are taken from reputable textbooks. All of them are true (in a way). All of them are determinist. None of them indicate the full picture.

The full picture is best illustrated by the findings in a large scale survey of patients with ulcerative colitis and Crohn's

disease carried out by the World Organization of Gastroenterology (Figure 3.4). It is true that giant cells and granulomata, where present, were almost exclusively found in cases
labelled as Crohn's disease. Only very occasionally were one
or two giant cells or granulomata found in patients subse-
quently classified as having ulcerative colitis. However,
much more importantly, although giant cells/granulomata
were highly suggestive of Crohn's disease *where present*,
only around 20% of cases with Crohn's disease actually had
evidence of these features on biopsy.

Look carefully at Figure 3.4 and then consider the information in the light of the 'determinist' textbook statement.
If you look carefully and think hard enough, you will be able
to work out why so many diagnoses of Crohn's disease are
missed, and why the 'lead time' between Crohn's disease
patients presenting to hospital and having their disease
diagnosed is well over one year in several studies. The
surgeon thinking along determinist lines will diagnose

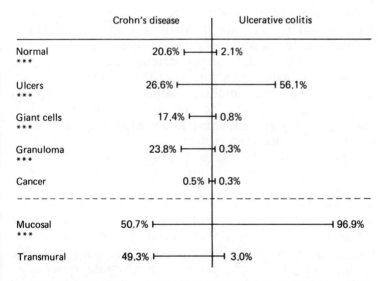

Figure 3.4 Biopsy findings concerning histopathological features in a large-scale
survey of patients with ulcerative colitis and Crohn's disease in numerous countries. (From Bouchier I A D and de Dombal F T (1979) *Scandinavian Journal of
Gastroenterology*; **14** (suppl. 56): 1–27).

Crohn's disease when giant cells and granulomata are present, and will diagnose ulcerative colitis (or some other condition) when they are absent. Now consider what this means in practice. If you *do* see giant cells and/or granulomata, you *will* diagnose Crohn's disease, and 19 times out of 20 you will be right. But what if you do *not* see giant cells or granulomata? Then presumably you will diagnose ulcerative colitis, and almost half the time you will be wrong.

If however, you are thinking along probabilistic lines you will have realized that whilst the *presence of these signs is a strong indicator (better than 20:1) for Crohn's disease, their absence is relatively meaningless.* You will have realized from the data in the figure that approximately three quarters of patients with Crohn's disease do not have these features on biopsy. So, if a patient has other features of Crohn's disease (such as segmental changes or patchy endoscopic findings, or maybe anorectal complications) you will consider diagnosing Crohn's disease *on the balance of probabilities.*

The balance of probabilities, like it or not, is what clinical decision making is all about. Many students have difficulty in coming to terms with this situation. It is so much easier to think in terms of determinist statements (giant cell plus granuloma equals Crohn's disease) that many students decide to opt for the simplicity. Some even have difficulty coming to terms with the concept of probability altogether. Surgeons, they reason, must know what they are doing, because they appear so certain.

If you fall into this category you are in good company. When presented with the probability theory of quantum mechanics, Einstein refused to accept it, and remarked famously, and (probably) erroneously, "God does not play dice with the universe". Professor Niels Bohr, the Danish atomic physicist, went further, declaring that a student who was not shocked by probability theory had not understood the theory in the first place. Indeed, probability theory as we shall see shortly can be very complex indeed, but for now it is important merely to re-emphasize that all is not 'black and white' in clinical medicine or surgery and that most diagnoses and decisions are made on the balance of probability rather than on certainty. If you aim for certainty of decision you will in most instances be disappointed. If you aim to make decisions on the balance of probabilities, then the laws of probability which drive the universe will be on your side and most of the time (by definition) you will be right.

Combining pieces of evidence and quantifying probability

There is one other aspect that we have not considered so far, and that is how and why pieces of evidence are combined. I have left this towards the end of the chapter, because in truth I think this is far less important than understanding the need to think in terms of probability and its theory. However, the way in which probability can be quantified has excited more interest amongst mathematicians than any other aspect of surgical decision making. So skip this section if you wish. For those who are interested however, I offer a brief introduction looking at the most popular of these methods, known as Bayes Theorem, in rather more detail.

Why we need to combine pieces of evidence should be obvious from the previous paragraphs. Consider two patients (both children) with suspected appendicitis whom you are called to see in the Emergency Room. Both have been seen by their family doctor. The first is said to have right lower quadrant pain *and* tenderness, the second merely to have right lower quadrant pain. Which is more likely to have appendicitis?

Of course the former, and if we now add the additional evidence that the patient has rebound tenderness and guarding in the same place, acute appendicitis becomes highly probable. But that is not the point here. The point is that we have arrived at a (highly probable) diagnosis by *combining items of evidence, none of which individually have the power of the combined picture.*

So the question is not *whether* we need to combine individual items of evidence like symptoms or signs (of course we do), but *how* this should be done. Over the years this question has evoked much effort, and involved much discussion (and no little controversy). Very early in the history of medicine, the need to combine clinical features was realized; and this was done in one of several ways.

The 'classical picture'

Many centuries ago (as far back, at least, as the Hippocratic system of medicine) it was realized that patients with the same underlying condition frequently presented in more or less the same way.

In ancient times, life was much simpler, partly because nobody knew the causation of disease. So swelling of the ankles and lower limbs was due to a disease called 'dropsy', defined as 'swelling of the ankles and lower limbs'. As understanding of disease processes increased, so did the complexity of the relationship between clinical appearances and underlying disease process. In particular, it was realized that:

- clinical symptoms or physical signs may have more than one cause
- disease processes may result in more than one clinical feature.

These problems were initially tackled in a simple and effective way, by developing the 'classical picture' of a particular disease, a collection of symptoms and signs which taken together were usually (but not always) present when a particular disease process was occurring. When all of them were present the case was said to be 'classical'; when most were present, and usually this was about two-thirds of the time, the case was said to be 'typical', and when few or none were present, the case was said to be 'atypical'.

This arrangement worked very well for centuries, and still does in many instances. You will find an excellent example on p. 74 relating to acute appendicitis – the more features listed in Figure 5.4 a patient exhibits, the more likely they are to have an acutely inflamed appendix. If they have *all* the features, the case is 'classical', if *most*, 'typical', and if *none* (which is very rare), 'atypical'. You will see that throughout this book I have recommended you should develop your own (similar) short-lists for various clinical problems. That is what your chief has already done; and it is a big help. So why use numbers?

So why use numbers?

Short-lists of 'classic' symptoms are fine in 'classical' or 'typical' cases. In totally 'atypical' cases, they are useless, but so is everything else. So why bother with numbers? Actually, there are quite a few reasons why many scientists (and an increasing proportion of clinicians) are interested in using numbers when combining clinical features in order to make a diagnostic (or prognostic) prediction.

First, in many given situations, not many patients are 'classic' cases, and only about half to two-thirds are 'typical'. These are the easy cases, and the rest may be fiendishly difficult. Second, medical data are 'soft', only rarely do any two observers record *exactly* the same data about a patient. Third, and most important, in *any* short list of features, some features, like the animals in George Orwell's farm, are more equal than others.

Think back to p. 35 and the data on granulomata and giant cells in Crohn's disease. We saw there that if these are *present*, Crohn's disease is highly likely, but their absence is meaningless. So, instead of a short-list that scored granuloma as $+1$, no granuloma as -1 (and so on) we can draw up a short-list that scores granuloma as $+27$ and giant cells as $+20$, and ignore their absence because it does not help. But why stop there? We can do this for *all* the important clinical, radiological, endoscopic, and histopathological appearances, add up the total at the end, and make a diagnostic prediction. (Actually, what we have just described is the Clamp/Softley OMGE Scoring System (Figure 3.5), which in worldwide tests agrees with experienced clinical opinion in 90–95% of cases.)

Bayes Theorem
Why stop there? Why not use the raw data (as in Figure 3.4) to produce not just an approximate score but an *exact*

WORLD ORGANISATION OF GASTROENTEROLOGY RESEARCH COMMITTEE

INFLAMMATORY BOWEL DISEASE

Scoring system to differentiate between ulcerative colitis and Crohn's disease

Age:		Blood:		Findings:	
0–19	+1	None	+6	Stenosis	+4
50–59	−1	Slight	−2	Ulcers	−1
70+	−2	+++	−5	Dilatation	+4
				Fistula	+6
Duration:		Mucus:		Skip lesions	+8
1–3 months	−2	None	+3		
3–6 months	−1	Slight	−1		
		+++	−2	Endoscopy:	
				Normal	+12
Family history:				Ulcers	−1
U. colitis	−2	Comps.:		Stenosis	+2
Crohn's disease	+4	Perianal	+7	Bleeding	−4
		Fistula	+8		
Past history:		Systemic	+1	Diffuse	−2
Appx.	+3			Patchy	+16
Anal fissure	+7	Nutrition:			
Fistula	+4	Emaciated	+2	Biopsy:	
None	−1			Normal	+5
		Tenderness:		Ulcers	−3
Site of pain:		R.L.Q.	+10	Giant cell	+20
R.L.Q.	+10	Upper half	−2	Granuloma	+27
L.L.Q.	−1	Left half	−3		
Right half	+2	Central	+6	Mucosal	−1
Left half	−6	None	−1	Transmural	+16
Central	+2				
No pain	−1	Abdominal findings:		Lab tests:	
		Distension	+2	Hb <10	−1
Type of pain:		Mass	+10	WBC 20 +	+1
Severe	+2			ALB. 5 +	−1
Steady	+2	Radiology:		Plats. < 150	−6
		Normal	−3	400 +	+1
Bowels:		Continuous	−1	Iron 20–40	+1
Normal	+1	Segmental	+11		
Diarrhoea x1/day	+3				
Diarrhoea x10/day	−2	Site:			
		Jejunum	+7		
		Ileum	+31		
		Right colon	+1		
		Left colon	−1		
		Rectum	−3		

Overall score: positive favours Crohns, negative favours ulcerative colitis

Figure 3.5 Scoring system for discrimination between patients with ulcerative colitis and Crohn's disease proposed by the Research Committee of the World Organization of Gastroenterology. (From Clamp S E, Myren L *et al.* (1982) *British Medical Journal*; **284**: 91–5.

probability? To accomplish this you need a computer to hold the raw data and perform the (tedious) maths, and you need an appropriate mathematical model. In short you need something like 'Bayes Theorem'.

The story of Bayes Theorem is an interesting and unusual one. The Reverend Thomas Bayes was an 18th century clergyman. He died in 1761, and you may still find his grave in Bunhill Fields (near Old Street underground station in London). Actually, although it is called Bayes Theorem, 'his' theorem was published 2 years later by a friend of his (the Reverend Richard Price) who 'found it' while clearing out Bayes' desk, or so he said.

For the historically minded it can still be found as "An essay towards solving a problem in the doctrine of chance" (1763) Philos Trans R Soc Lond, **53**, 370–418. For the rest of us, 200 years on, it is difficult to unravel who said what, which bits were written by whom, and as you can see from the page numbers, the paper does go on a bit. However, in all of this some quite crucial concepts emerge, which are very relevant indeed to the practice of clinical medicine:

- prior probability
- conditional probability
- final probability.

Now, of course, Bayes never talked about clinical medicine (he was trying to prove the existence of God by assessing the probability the sun would rise in the East next day). But the concepts of moving from prior probability, through conditional probability, to a final probability are so important that we must understand them if we are to understand how surgeons (and others) analyse information.

Prior Probability implies starting probability. It implies what the odds are from general experience before you know anything about the particular case.

As you learn more, each new item of information carries its own weight of evidence. This new evidence alters (or *conditions*) your original (or prior) estimates. So the weight of evidence which each new item of information carries, is called its *conditional probability*.

Gradually, as you obtain each item of evidence, your starting point (prior probability) is modified more and more by the total weight of evidence from each item – until there are no more new items to add. All the evidence is in, and at this point you finish up with what is known as a posterior or *final probability*.

Let us take a leaf out of Bayes' book, and illustrate each of these with a bizarre example. Imagine you are standing in the middle of a large field and behind you, you hear hoof-beats. You naturally want to know the cause, but unfortunately there is a thick fog. So what is behind you?

Before you reply 'no idea', that is nonsense. You actually have quite a good idea. You have the *prior probabilities*. You know that to generate hoof-beats an animal must have hooves. On the basis of prior probability, therefore, you expect to see (eventually) possibly a horse or a cow, because these are common animals. You might expect to see a zebra or a water buffalo, but these would not come high on your list because they are not common.

That is all that prior probability implies, except that Bayes goes a little further and points out that if you knew the total population of horses/cows/whatever in your part of the world you could put an exact figure to the prior probability of each. If, for example, you knew where you were, knew the farmer who owned the field, and knew (from him) that he had about 100 cows and half a dozen horses, you could estimate (even without seeing the animal in question) there was about a 20:1 chance the animal was a cow. That is all that prior probability implies.

Bayes Theorem, however, goes on to suggest that these 'prior' probabilities are altered or 'conditioned' by extra evidence before you arrive at a 'final' probability. Suppose, for example, as the mist clears, you can now see a large sign in the field that reads "Welcome to our Safari Park" and a companion, looking over your shoulder, informs you that the animal has stripes. You would (if you are wise) use these extra items of information to 'condition' your first prior estimates. Your 'final' notion might well be that in all probability you were being approached by a zebra.

Note that Bayes Theorem says 'in all probability'. Your companion might (having seen the sign) be joking. It might be worse, you might be in the process of being attacked by a rhinoceros but *on the balance of probability*, a zebra is most likely. Note also that I have left out a number of mathematical issues – how the probabilities were combined together, the precise final estimates and so on. They do not matter here. What matters is that you get a clear idea of how we can use the *principles* of Bayes Theorem to solve medical problems.

So let us forget safari parks and zebras, and turn to a clinical problem. Let us think again about the situation we faced in Figure 3.4 and the surrounding text. We have a patient with inflammatory bowel disease (IBD); and we want to decide, whether we are dealing with ulcerative colitis (UC) or with Crohn's disease (CD). Figure 3.6 shows you how Bayes Theorem works it out, by comparing a 'new' case, item by item, with 1 000 other 'known' cases. To start with our prior probabilities (the prevalences in the centre in question) are 60UC:40CD. Bayes merely reflects this. After these 'prior' probabilities have been 'conditioned' by the interview and examination, the picture is still pretty even, though some items (perianal complications, severe pain) have begun to swing the probability a little in favour of Crohn's disease. However, when we add in the investigation data (normal endoscopy, segmental disease, ileal disease, skip lesions) the balance of probability comes down very heavily in favour of Crohn's disease.

Note that (as in the safari park) we can never be certain and nor can Bayes Theorem. The patient may not have IBD at all. The patient may be lying. But, on balance, *if* the patient has IBD and *if* the information is correct, your verdict, and that of Bayes Theorem, would be that Crohn's disease is highly likely. As high as 99% likely? – perhaps not, but it does not matter. The important ideas to take from this discussion are as follows:

● matters are rarely absolute in clinical decision
● often no one symptom, sign or test is pathognomonic

CASE REF.

FEMALE	X.RAY: DISEASE SEGMENTAL
AGE 0–19 YEARS.	. . . . SITE: + ILEUM
DURATION 3–6 MTHS.	. . . . SITE: + R.COLON
NO RELEVANT FAMILY HISTORY	. . . . SITE: + L. COLON
NO RELEVANT PAST HISTORY	. . . . ULCERS
SITE OF PAIN: LOWER HALF	. . . . SKIP LESIONS
SLIGHT PAIN	NORMAL ENDOSCOPY
INTERMITTENT PAIN	NORMAL BIOPSY
BOWELS: DIARRHOEA	Hb. 10
. . . . x 5–10	WBC. 10
. . . . NO BLOOD	ALB. 3–5
. . . . NO MUCUS	ESR. 40+
NO PERIANAL COMPLICATIONS	PL. 150–400
NO OTHER FISTULA	IRON 20–40
NO SYSTEMIC COMPLICATIONS	
TEMPERATURE 37–37.9°C	
PULSE 80–99	
NUTRITION: EMACIATED	
NO ABDOMINAL TENDERNESS	
NO ABDOMINAL DISTENTION	
NO ABDOMINAL MASS	

Crohn's	Colitis	Crohn's	Colitis
79.35	20.64	99.99	0.00

Figure 3.6 Illustration of the basic principles underlying Bayes Theorem for both non-medical and clinical situations. Note that the prior probability is about 50:50. Note that the clinical picture conditions this in favour of Crohn's disease (80:20) and the investigations to the point where the final probability of Crohn's disease is (almost) 100%.

- there is a need to combine information
- you cannot do this without a pencil, a (big) sheet of paper and a lot of time and effort (or a computer to save the drudgery)
- you can, however, follow the principles involved. You can get in the habit of starting with prior probabilities, 'conditioning' these by additional data and arriving not at a certainty but at a balance of probabilities, which will be right more often than not
- to do this, you need to develop 'short lists' of features for each clinical situation – half a dozen or so – those which will do most to reduce your uncertainty and help you towards a correct diagnosis and decision.

Practical implications

All of this talk of data analysis and probability theory is (sometimes only vaguely!) appreciated by almost every medical student after a month or so on the surgical wards. Unfortunately most students do not follow through and think about the implications for their clinical practice after qualification and also for their study at undergraduate and postgraduate level. So in the final section of this chapter, let us look through some of the practical implications of what we have discussed and see how you can make use of them both in study and in routine clinical practice.

1. Define your objectives. Remember that there is more to the surgical decision than merely tying a label on a patient. In weighing the evidence therefore, you should keep in the forefront of your mind the objectives and the questions you are trying to answer, including:

- do you believe the evidence from the patient?
- what is the patient's main problem?
- what is the disease process causing the problem?
- how severe and how active is the disease?
- are there any complicating conditions or issues?

2. Know your limitations. The next practical implication of the discussion on previous pages involves a knowledge of the limitations that we all face in analysing information. On the one hand it is unlikely that a single piece of evidence (symptom or sign) will lead you irrevocably to a diagnosis and decision. On the other hand, it is impossible to analyse at once all the information you have collected. The most likely situation is that a combination of symptoms and signs will be found somewhere in the case history, which together allow a sensible diagnosis and decision to be made and taken.

What you should therefore do is to train yourself to look in each case history for that critical half dozen or so features on which the decision is going to be based.

3. Know the weight of evidence.   In order to weigh up the evidence appropriately, however, you need to know what weight should be attached to each item. Otherwise, you have little chance of selecting your half dozen or so critical features that will lead you to the correct management of the patient.

The problem of course is you do not know what these 'short lists' are; your chief does (and uses them) but you do not, and thus cannot follow his example. Herein lies a problem, which has crucial implications in terms of making the best of your education. Next time you are on the wards, and you come across a disease you are not familiar with, or a patient who does not present with the 'classical' picture, ask yourself a simple question. If you were only able to obtain six or seven items of information *and no more*, which would be the ones to choose? If you do this sensibly (and you may need to consult both your chief and more than one textbook) you should have your 'short list'. It may not be perfect, but it will serve you until you develop your own experience.

4. Play the probabilities. I regularly take with me into decision making seminars a large overhead transparency of Omar Sharif playing cards. I use this when some student whose mind has been wandering is asked to supply a diagnostic prediction, and mentions some gross rarity such as 'porphyria' or 'polycythaemia'. The unfortunate student, asked would you wager £100 that the most lateral card in Mr. Sharif's hand is the ace of spades, invariably declines (the odds are 51 to 1 against). Asked, 'why then have you just wagered the patient's life on a probability 100 times less likely than the one for which you just turned down a wager of £100?' students become defensive, argumentative or embarrassed, but they get the point. I am not in favour of hectoring or embarrassing students, but they (and you) must understand it is no use knowing the probabilities unless you play the probabilities.

5. Don't be 'brilliant'. There has to be a first time for everything, and you probably find an exhortation *not* to be brilliant is unusual. So let me repeat it: do not, repeat, do not be 'brilliant'. The 'brilliant' decision maker is the one who (just occasionally, and often quite by chance) gets right an obscure case. People talk about it for days. In extreme circumstances, it rates a case report in a medical journal. The 'solid plodder' on the other hand, is one who does the simple things, does them well, has a good *overall* track record, and who rarely misses out on a straightforward case or a common condition.

This is what you should aim for, not occasional brilliance. In weighing up the evidence, define your objectives, know your limitations, know the weight of evidence, know the probabilities, and play the probabilities. You will not get into the medical literature once every 10 years, and no one will name a syndrome after you, but your patients will thank you for it.

4

Decision making: formal analysis versus clinical hunch

Sometimes, once you have elicited the clinical features from the patient and have analysed these features in the way described in previous chapters, it will be blindingly obvious what decision should be made and what course of action taken – sometimes, but not always. Some decision theorists would even argue not very often. Remember it is uncertainty that characterizes surgical decisions, and distinguishes them from the classification of rocks, flowers or trees. Only rarely will you be absolutely certain of the best course of action for a particular patient. More frequently, you will need (on the basis of correct and appropriately analysed evidence) to make a decision when there is still some element of doubt as to what to do for the best.

Until recently, as we saw in Chapter 1, surgical decision making was governed by 'rules', 'aphorisms', or 'intuition', and defended (when wrong) by involving the concept of clinical freedom. Until recently, virtually all such decisions could be defended by invoking this concept, usually in a sentence beginning "In my clinical judgement". This is no longer the case, and there have been a number of animated discussions concerning the whole concept of clinical freedom. On the whole the public seems to have sided with the views of Professor Hampton who wrote in the early 1980s "Clinical freedom is dead... and we need not mourn its passing". Personally, I prefer the slightly more gentle views expressed by the Rev. Gordon Dunstan (1986) who pointed out that clinical freedom is still a valid concept. However, it is not a right but a privilege granted by society to the surgeon in the expectation that the surgeon will utilize all his/her best efforts for the benefit of the patient.

This has led to the concept of an 'ideal' surgical decision – one that follows logically from an appropriate analysis of impeccably collected information from the patient, a decision which is easy to understand, easy to explain and easy to justify both to the patient and society if the decision turns out to be wrong.

However, as John Clarke has remarked in his tutorial series on surgical decision making, 'whereas ideally all medical decisions are logical conclusions from the facts, in reality they are not! Medical decisions invariably are estimates of probabilities and trade offs, and unfortunately people (even experts) make errors in estimating the probabilities and balancing the trade-offs'.

What John Clarke says is important. He re-emphasizes the uncertainties involving surgical decision making and the need in making such decisions to constantly (as he puts it) 'balance the trade offs'. This situation has led over the years to a considerable amount of research, which has in the main taken two forms. First, research workers have studied how doctors and particularly surgeons make decisions in practice (this branch of research is known generally as 'process tracing'). Second, perhaps because of criticisms about the 'mystique' of clinical medicine, attempts have been made to formalize surgical decision making, and the literature involving 'formal decision analysis' in clinical medicine is now very extensive indeed.

In theory, formal decision analysis applied to surgical problems is extremely valuable. It makes decision making 'logical', easy to understand, easy to explain, and yields valuable insights into the process by which surgeons make decisions. However, formal decision analysis is as yet a very young science, and there is an additional problem in clinical surgery. For the worst outcome of all would be for surgeons to become obsessed with formal decision analysis to the point where they found it difficult to make decisions at all. This is not entirely fanciful. You may remember the ancient fable of Dionysius and his ass – the poor animal starved to death when placed equidistant between two equally inviting piles of hay and was unable to make a decision as to which direction to move in.

Nevertheless, decision analysis has an immense future, and raises a number of important questions concerning practical surgical decision making. So in the next few sections, we shall look at formal decision analysis and its potential. We shall also look at the problems associated with formal decision analysis, and finally, look at how all of this can help us in the practical day to day situations in clinical surgery.

The power and potential of formal decision analysis

Let us imagine that you are dealing with a patient whom you have interviewed and examined thoroughly. You have weighed up all the evidence correctly and appropriately, and now you have to make a decision as to whether to operate on the patient or not. The disease is immaterial. It may be a suspected appendicitis, cancer, or indeed any other condition for which surgery is appropriate. Should you operate or not?

The textbooks are often not much help here. The textbooks will merely tell you that the treatment for appendicitis or cancer (or whatever), is 'operation'. The problem is *you do not know* whether the patient does or does not have the condition in question. Nevertheless, despite this uncertainty, a decision must be made whether or not to operate.

The concepts of utility and probability

Decision theory jargon refers to this situation (which is the simplest we can construct) as a 'two by two decision table'. That is to say there are really only two choices, and each of these two choices can be either right or wrong, as illustrated in Figure 4.1. This figure, the first step in formal decision analysis, offers no guidance. It merely sets out the alternatives, and the consequences of each decision (right or wrong). To offer formal guidance we need to look at two further concepts. One we have met before (the concept of probability) and one needs to be introduced now, because it is a difficult concept and has caused much argument over the last 20 years. This concept is the concept of 'utility'.

	Decision	
	Operate	Do not operate
Appendicitis	correct	possible perforation
No appendicitis	unnecessary operation	correct

Figure 4.1 Two-way decision table showing possible outcomes of alternative forms of therapy in patients with suspected appendicitis.

What is 'utility'?

We are getting into some deep water here, so let us first consider what we mean by 'utility'. The dictionary definition of the word 'utility' includes the synonym 'usefulness'. Of course this is reasonable, and it is appropriate here. We all went into medicine in the hope of doing some good to patients. Fine, but how is this vague notion of doing good to be assessed? Can we quantify it in some way to enable us to say *how much* good we have done? It sounds an odd concept, but there are various ways of doing this. One way, for example, is to work out how much people (or governments) are prepared to pay to have a particular treatment available. Another way (and some would argue a better way) is to consider the *outcome* of a treatment, and how much the patient likes and values that (outcome) state of health.

That is all 'utility' means. Clarke (1990) defines 'utility' as a term used to describe the subjective worth of an outcome to a particular person. It is a measure of peoples' preferences and it incorporates both psychological values and personal values as well as mathematical values. This means in practice that whatever the doctor does, and whatever the outcome for the patient, then that particular outcome will have a particular value for the patient; and we call that value to the patient, its 'utility'. Note incidentally that we are talking here about the value to the *patient*. The same procedure may have a different perceived utility to others. Different persons see matters in different lights. Happiness, as the song says, means different things to different people.

But this is not the fault of utility theory. All that the concept of 'utility' does is to assign a mathematical value to each of these outcomes, usually on a scale extending from 0 to 1. The 0 end of the scale represents the worst possible outcome (usually the patient's death) and in contrast the value 1 on the scale represents the best possible outcome imaginable (such as a completely painless recovery to full health and vigour). However, as we can see from Figure 4.2, there are other possible outcomes, and each of these outcomes can be given a 'utility' in the same way. Clearly, the 'utility' of the intermediate outcome should lie somewhere between 0 and 1 and to illustrate the way in which any decision (e.g. to operate or not) can be formalized we merely assign values to each of the various outcomes along the lines set out in Figure 4.2.

How do we decide upon 'utility' values?
To do this, let us go back again to the situation in Figure 4.1. Let us look at each of the possible outcomes in turn and assign an arbitrary 'utility' to them (Figure 4.3). First, which is the best outcome? Which outcome would you prefer if you were a patient? Personally I would opt for number 4 – where I did not have appendicitis, I did not have an operation and I went home the next day perfectly well. This would be the

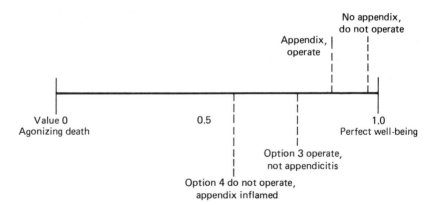

Figure 4.2 Same situation as Figure 4.1, but presented as decision 'tree' with utilities for the various outcomes.

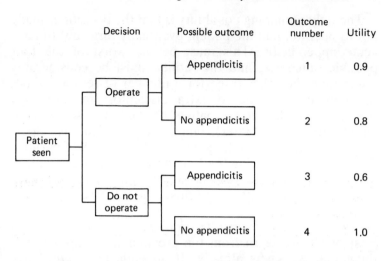

Decision	Possible outcome	Outcome number	Utility
Appendicitis	1	0.9
No appendicitis	2	0.8
Appendicitis	3	0.6
No appendicitis	4	1.0

Figure 4.3 Same analysis as in Figure 4.1 and 4.2, but with utilities attached to each outcome.

best outcome and so we can assign a 'utility' to it – a 'utility' of 1.

What would be the next best outcome? Probably the reverse of the coin. The decision to operate *was* made, an acute appendicitis *was* found, and a full recovery ensued. What 'utility' should be assigned to this? Clearly it cannot be 1 because the patient has experienced the trauma and discomfort of an operation; but clearly it cannot be far away from 1 because the correct treatment has been administered and the patient has made a complete recovery. For the sake of the present argument we will assign a 'utility' of 0.9 to this outcome.

There is of course a third alternative – the decision to operate is made but no appendicitis or other surgical condition is found (a negative laparotomy). What is the 'utility' of this condition? Clearly it cannot be 1 because the patient has undergone an operation. Equally clearly, it cannot be as high as 0.9, because the operation was unnecessary. For the purposes of our discussion we will assign a 'utility' to this outcome of 0.8.

The only remaining possibility is that the decision is made not to operate, and the patient eventually turns out to have acute appendicitis. This must be the worst of the four possible outcomes, and the 'utility' must be considerably lower than the other three for a number of reasons. First, the patient has suffered extra discomfort for hours or possibly days. Second the patient has had the discomfort of an operation (albeit later). Finally, and particularly important, the patient has undergone considerable risk of perforation (needlessly) during the time period of the delay before operation. For these reasons we may assign an arbitrary value of 0.6 to the 'utility' of this final outcome.

Using 'utilities' for formal decision analysis
First of all, we learn from the previous paragraphs something that we knew already. If appendicitis is *absolutely certain*, it is better to operate (utility 0.9) than not to operate (utility 0.6). Conversely, if appendicitis is *not possible*, it is better not to operate (utility 1) than to operate (utility 0.8). However, the problem is that we do not know whether the patient has appendicitis or not. All we can do is to assign a probability (p) to this, so that the patient has a probability (p) of appendicitis and therefore a probability (1 minus p) of not having appendicitis.

We are now in a position to illustrate *formally* this clinical decision. As already pointed out, the doctor has two alternatives (first to operate, second not to operate). According to decision theory the doctor should choose which alternative has the highest 'utility' to the patient. You may think this is just a fancy way of saying what the Hippocratic oath said several thousand years ago. You would be right. However, decision theory allows us to say this with a little more precision than Hippocrates. For the 'combined utility' to the patient of each choice amounts to the sum of the 'utilities' of the two outcomes of that choice multiplied in each case by the probability of that outcome occurring. Therefore in mathematical terms, the 'utility' of operating (which we shall call U_{op}) can be written:

$$U_{op} = P_a U_1 + (1-P_a)U_2$$

where P_a is the probability of the patient having appendicitis, and U_1 is the 'utility' of outcome 1, in Figure 4.1. Similarly,

$$U_{nop} = P_aU_3 + (1-P_a)U_4$$

Sorry about these equations. Generally speaking, I hate equations: I have included these two because they are simple and powerful. We have already seen what happens if the surgeon is sure. What these two equations now allow us to construct is a graph (Figure 4.4) for each level of probability (i.e. the estimated probability that the patient has appendicitis).

Suppose for example that you are completely unsure and that the probability of appendicitis or non-surgical disease is 50:50. What should the surgeon do? In fact you can do the mathematics yourself quite easily by looking at Figure 4.4

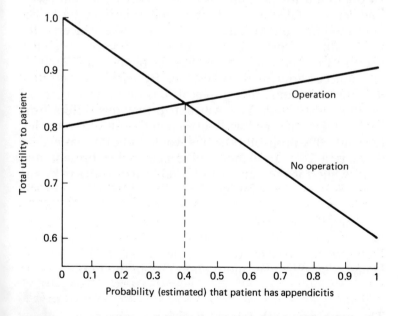

Figure 4.4 Graphic illustration of the utility to patient of (a) operating and (b) not operating for each level of probability when the patient actually does have appendicitis.

and the two equations. I suspect you will find the value of operating amounts to $(0.5 \times 0.9) + (0.5 \times 0.8) = 0.85$. You will also find that the value of not operating amounts to $(0.5 \times 0.6) + (0.5 \times 1) = 0.8$.

Our formal analysis of the problem therefore indicates that, if absolutely unsure, the surgeon should operate, because the overall 'utility' to the patient (bearing in mind that the surgeon may be wrong) is higher after operation. Indeed, on the basis of this analysis, our formal graph indicates that if the doctor is more than about 40% sure the patient has appendicitis then an operation should be carried out.

This simple diagram in Figure 4.4 is quite crucial to any understanding of decision theory in medicine. Here we have applied it to a relatively simple problem, but it can be applied (at least in theory) to any medical or surgical problem, however complex. For example, we can consider an operation for possible cancer in exactly the same way. The decision table is exactly the same as in Figure 4.1. The only modification we have needed to make concerns the utility for outcome 3 (not operating, cancer present), because the vast majority of these patients will eventually die unnecessarily of their disease. By simple substitution into the equations, the graphical illustration in Figure 4.5 can be constructed. You will notice that this differs from Figure 4.4 in that the 'break-even point' is moved to the left (around 20% probability). This would indicate that even if there is a 20% probability of cancer being present it is worthwhile for the patient to be subjected to the risks and discomfort of an operation.

The preceding paragraphs, therefore, illustrate (albeit in a very simple fashion) the general application of the principles of formal decision analysis. It should by now be clear that these principles have a considerable amount to offer and are likely to become ever more important in the future.

The problems with formal decision analysis

Many surgeons are fearful of formal decision analysis, sometimes for reasons which I personally find less than

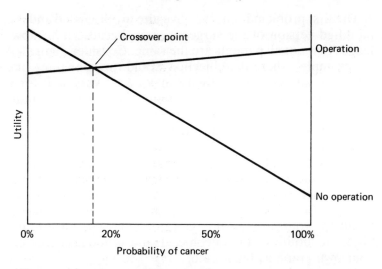

Figure 4.5 Same analysis as Figure 4.4, but for a patient with suspected cancer and a very low utility for option 3: cancer, do not operate. Note how different utilities shift 'break-even' point to the left.

satisfactory. They argue that formal decision analysis such as that outlined above is all very well but it fails to take into account 'imponderable' factors concerning the patient, which the 'experienced' surgeon automatically assesses. Each patient, it is argued, is an individual and needs to be treated on a purely individual basis. This comes close to pleading the 'mystique' of clinical medicine or surgery, and has been rather neatly countered by Lorenz, who argues that from the patient's viewpoint, the patient attends the surgeon with precisely the opposite in mind. That is to say the patient attends an experienced surgeon rather than a novice precisely because the patient hopes the experienced surgeon *has* seen the problem before and knows what to do about it.

There are however, a number of really quite severe problems with formal decision analysis – at least as it is currently understood or practised. These may be overcome in the future but at the moment they represent a considerable obstacle to the routine use of formal decision theory throughout clinical practice.

The first problem is one we have already discussed and is a modified version of the surgeons' fear, because it acknowledges that not all patients are the same. Consider Figure 4.4 for example, where the objection would run something like this. The analysis in the figure may be all very well for a typical fit young patient, but supposing the patient was unfit, or old, or suffered from some other disease (such as haemophilia), which would increase the risk of operation, then the 'utility' values for the different treatments and outcomes would be greatly changed.

This is clearly a problem though it is not an insuperable one. It merely implies that the 'utility' values need to be changed for individual patients. (You may care to experiment for yourself with the data in Figure 4.4, substituting different 'utilities' for outcomes 1 and 4 and constructing your own graph as Figure 4.6.)

There are however, at least two further problems. The first concerns the values attached to p (the probability of disease). We have blithely assumed that the doctor's own estimates of probability can be used for this purpose, but

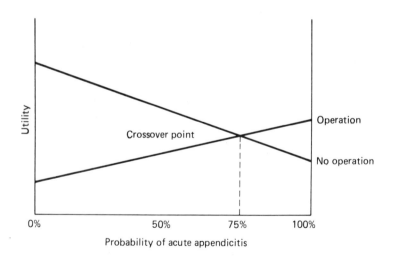

Figure 4.6 Same analysis as Figure 4.4 and 4.5, but for a patient with suspected appendicitis who is unfit, old and suffering from other, multiple, severe diseases. Very low utility for option 3: operate, not appendicitis.

studies have shown that doctors are highly fallible in this respect. The profound effect this might have is obvious. For example, a number of studies have shown that when doctors intuitively rate the chance of appendicitis as '50:50', only about one quarter of patients actually turn out to have appendicitis. So should 25% or 50% be specified for the value of p?

Even this problem can be overcome (by using estimates of probability based on large series of real life patients). There is however a final obstacle. This last obstacle, by far the most formidable, concerns the assigning of values to the 'utilities' of the various outcomes of different modes of treatment. For example, if we return to the situation illustrated in Figure 4.4, we might all agree that the utility of outcome 1 and outcome 4 are (probably) reasonably well assessed. The utilities we have assigned to outcomes 2 and 3 (unnecessary operation and missing appendicitis, respectively) are, by contrast, highly debatable; and it is quite impossible to give a global figure, which will be appropriate for every patient. For example, we know from experience that rupture of the appendix increases the mortality (by a factor of 5 to 10) and we might argue that this can easily be allowed for in assigning a 'utility'. Things become more complicated however, when we realize that the chance of rupture of the appendix in a case of missed appendicitis varies from 3% in a young adult male to 30% in a small child or elderly person.

Possibly even this could be allowed for (albeit with some difficulty); but what value should we assign to an 'unnecessary' operation? To a young healthy adult male, an unnecessary operation might not matter very much. The risk is small, an appendix scar no great handicap, and the removal of a normal appendix might seem to be of negligible importance – in some cases even quite welcome as a prophylactic measure, particularly if the patient intends to travel to remote parts of the world. Others, however, would feel quite differently. A young girl concerned about her appearance, an old person with chronic obstructive airways disease, or the occasional unfortunate patient who suffers massive intra-abdominal sepsis following negative laparotomy might all have considerably different views about the 'negligible harm' done by this simple procedure.

It is this difficulty, the representation of the patient's 'feelings' in mathematical terms, which constitutes the biggest obstacle to the widespread introduction of all decision analysis into clinical medicine. A number of studies have addressed this problem, often using what are known as wagering techniques (e.g. how much money would you be prepared to pay to avoid such and such an outcome) and undoubtedly in the future the infant science of formal decision analysis in clinical surgery will be much refined. However, the difficulties in assigning probabilities, and above all 'utilities', to patient outcomes represent a formidable obstacle to be overcome.

The practical value of formal decision analysis

It is tempting to conclude from the previous paragraphs that formal decision analysis is an interesting topic, a complicated one, but one that has little to offer. In my view such a conclusion would be erroneous. There are a number of areas in which formal decision analysis has had an impact and is ever more likely to do so.

For example, the sort of formal decision analysis we have just discussed may not be appropriate to each and every individual patient, but it may well be appropriate in discussing *strategy for groups of patients*. Indeed it can be argued that formal decision analysis had it been performed in the past would have prevented some operations from ever being undertaken. Consider, for example, the situation in Figure 4.4 and think about other situations. Consider Figure 4.4 not in relation to appendicectomies but in relation to two different types of therapy for early breast cancer – lumpectomy and super-radical mastectomy. You may care to perform your own similar analysis of this issue by substituting various 'utilities' into the equation (using for p values the probability of surviving 5 years, and for U values the utility that you imagine the patient would put on each specific outcome).

I do not know what values you will choose. I do however, suspect very strongly that one of two conclusions will emerge. If you are to recommend super-radical mastectomy (*under any circumstances*) you will have to make one of two basic assumptions. Either, (i) women do not mind very much whether they undergo a minor or a major mutilating procedure; or (ii) the probability of 5-year survival following super-radical mastectomy is about 50% higher than following lumpectomy. Neither of these assumptions is valid, because both have been disproved by large scale studies. Consequently, you would have difficulty in these circumstances recommending super-radical mastectomy to any woman. Yet this operation was performed for decades as a routine procedure.

You may by now feel that had formal decision analysis been around at the time, super-radical mastectomy could never have been devised, or much less widely adopted, as a surgical procedure. If so, you have begun to glimpse the power of formal decision analysis in surgery and its value in assessing different therapeutic strategies.

Perhaps the greatest achievement however, of formal decision analysis is precisely that which is implied in the title. This type of analysis may yet not be all that appropriate for an individual patient. It is however, appropriate for looking at the way in which decisions are made in groups of patients. Indeed it gives us an extremely powerful tool, which has had a number of fascinating spin-offs. For example, by substituting into the equations not our own assessment of the 'utilities' but each individual surgeon's assessment of the 'utilities', we can get some information about the way that surgeon's mind is working. Similarly, we can gain a comparable impression of the way the patient is thinking by substituting a patient's values (which are quite different from the surgeon's values) into the equations. This has led incidentally to a whole new concept in patient values, that of the Quality Adjusted Life Year (QUALY), which is dealt with in more detail elsewhere (see p. 154); and by which we can gain new insights into the effect of various advances in therapy.

Practical implications

We have spent a considerable amount of time looking at
formal methods of surgical decision making – a topic which
some people might consider abstract, or even obscure – and
you may well be wondering how all this may help in your
own clinical practice. In fact it is of considerable practical
importance, because unless you understand how decisions
are made you are unlikely to make good decisions (other
than on a fortuitous basis). So we shall close this chapter
with a few suggestions that you can put into practice and
which should help you improve your own decision making
on a day to day basis.

1. Know what decision you are supposed to be making. Over
the years I have from time to time been disappointed to
observe a member of the Accident and Emergency department junior staff agonizing over a decision as to whether a
patient has acute appendicitis or a perforated duodenal
ulcer. Actually, in this situation it does not matter. They
both belong on the surgical wards and that is the decision
which should be made. Equally, I am disappointed when I
find a young surgeon on the wards agonizing over a decision
as to whether or not (yet another) blood test should be
performed in a patient with suspected appendicitis. That is
not the decision to be made. The patient should either be
taken to theatre or not. Therefore, the first step is to know
what *is* the relevant decision at a particular point in time,
and concentrate on getting *that* right.

2. Know your options. One of the main problems that
students and young doctors encounter in difficult situations
is they tend to think in terms of 'what shall I do?' instead of
thinking more constructively in terms of 'what options have I
got, and which one should I select'? The latter is far more
constructive, and a major step along the way to making
appropriate decisions (as on pp. 121 and 130) is a review of all
possible options, and a selection of the most appropriate one
from this option list.

3. Review possible outcomes and their consequences. I am not suggesting here that you should sit in the side ward and construct a decision table as in Figure 4.4 for each patient you see. However, as part of your review of the options, you would be wise, *en route* to making an appropriate decision, to consider (for each option) the possible outcomes and what will happen to the patient if that outcome occurs.

For an obvious example, consider Figure 4.5. I do not suggest that you make up such a mathematical table each time you see a patient with suspected cancer. You would be wise however, to learn that whilst over-caution may result in a negative investigation, overconfidence (sending the patient away without investigation at all) may lead to loss of life.

4. Review the patient's wishes. Once again I do not suggest that you embroil yourself in a detailed study of patient 'utility'. You would nevertheless be wise to learn from the discussion on p. 112 that the patient's wishes matter, and you would be wise in making your decision to involve the patient in the process as much as possible.

5. Review your own competence. In discussing the consequences of each option, you would also be wise to remember that there is sometimes a difference between the outcome as described in the textbooks (after operation by a highly experienced surgeon) and the possible outcome after an operation by yourself (never having attempted the procedure before). This may seem obvious, but unfortunately it is not so. Many of the problems encountered in clinical surgery stem from inexperienced young surgeons getting out of their depth and only calling for help when it is far too late (see p. 103). So remember, in selecting your option, bear in mind your own level of competence and what you can and cannot comfortably manage.

6. Make your decision. So to sum up the steps to be taken, which in essence are extremely simple, and include:

- know what decision you are making
- list the options available to you
- review the outcomes and consequences of each option
- exclude inappropriate options
- select the most appropriate option
- make your decision and act on it

Remember that it is this focus on decision making that particularly marks a surgeon from other clinical colleagues and if you are one of those people who finds it intensely difficult to make a decision, you may wish to think again about your proposed career in surgery. So by all means make your decision on the best possible information. Make your decision after the most appropriate analysis you can manage, and make your decision after consideration of all the features in the previous paragraphs, but make your decision and institute the necessary action.

7. Keep the patient informed. One final point before we leave this subject. Make your decision, and then tell the patient. Tell the patient what you propose to do, and tell the patient why you propose to do this. It is no longer appropriate (if indeed it ever was) to treat the patient as some kind of experimental subject participating in a process too difficult for them to understand. Patients at all times deserve the best information you can give them. If you doubt this, think back to the last time you were in an aeroplane, things were not going very well, and the pilot did not keep you fully informed. Remember your own irritation and apprehension, and consider the relative risks of flying in a civil aeroplane and undergoing an operative procedure. Remember that the biggest single complaint brought forward by consumers of all types (patients, passengers, whoever) is that they are not kept informed about what is happening. So tell the patient what you are doing, tell them why, and if you cannot tell them why, ask yourself whether you should be doing it in the first place.

Surgical decision making in practice: acute abdominal pain

So far we have spoken of decision making in a somewhat abstract sense. This is appropriate; we have already discussed the need for young surgeons to understand what the decision making process is all about, what the problems are in making surgical decisions, and the basic structure of how we arrive at surgical decisions. The time has now come to put these principles into practice.

So in this chapter we are going to discuss a particular situation and look at how the principles discussed in previous chapters apply to routine surgical practice. We are going to look at a patient with *acute abdominal pain*, because in most industrialized countries (and also in the tropics) this is the commonest surgical emergency and accounts for around about 1% of all admissions to hospital. However, the principles that underlie the *modus operandi* outlined in this chapter apply right across the board to all other surgical decisions, and this discussion should be seen, therefore, as something of a 'template' for all surgical decisions that you will need to make.

In this and subsequent chapters we are going to discuss general problems in the light of specific clinical 'vignettes' – brief clinical scenarios, which will be only too familiar to all surgeons of any experience. In respect of the acute abdomen, perhaps the commonest problem a young, inexperienced surgeon will routinely face runs along the following lines:

You are on duty on the surgical ward of a district general hospital. Late in the evening, you are asked to go to the Emergency Room to deal with a 15-year-old boy who has arrived there with his mother complaining of acute abdominal pain of 36 h duration. It is snowing, the telephone lines are down and you can expect no help from anybody more senior. You are entirely on your own. How do you proceed to sort out the patient's problem?

1. What do you need to know?

Before discussing details of patient management, it is worth-while at this point to step back for a moment and ask yourself what do you need to know in order to deal with the patient's problem? A suggested list of items is outlined in Figure 5.1. This figure is important for two reasons. First, if you are unfamiliar with or ignorant of any of the items in Figure 5.1 you are most unlikely to be able to make a sensible or appropriate decision. Second, and perhaps even more important, because Figure 5.1 outlines the type of information that a student or young surgeon needs to acquire about a particular medical or surgical problem in order to deal with it appropriately. Figure 5.1 is important in terms of both undergraduate and postgraduate self educa-tion. It represents (for each area of clinical medicine) what you need to know, and hence what you need to learn, in order to manage situations and solve patients' problems for them. Let us now deal with these items in turn.

1. What is acute abdominal pain?
2. Common causes
3. What questions to ask?
4. What examination to perform?
5. How to recognize common causes of pain (e.g. appendicitis)?
6. What to do?

Figure 5.1 Information needed to deal effectively with a patient suffering from acute abdominal pain.

2. What is acute abdominal pain?

Thinking back to Chapter 4, in order to sort out the patient's problem you need to know what the problem is. If you do not know what acute abdominal pain is, you are unlikely to get much further or make a sensible decision – because when dealing with acute abdominal pain the experienced surgeon will immediately think of a number of common causes (such as appendicitis), but if the particular patient does not have acute abdominal pain, then a whole range of other diagnoses and decisions may come into play. It is therefore, important to be clear at the outset what we mean by acute abdominal pain.

Acute abdominal pain (in most surgeons' opinions) implies presentation of a patient (to hospital in this instance) suffering from hitherto undiagnosed abdominal pain of less than 7–10 days duration.

Two elements of this definition are important. First the time frame. Beyond about 7 to 10 days you should be wary of categorizing a patient as having an 'acute abdomen' because if the patient has had pain for several weeks or a month or two, the list of possible diagnoses is completely different. Also the words 'hitherto undiagnosed' are important. Occasionally, a patient will present with an obvious and massive inguinal hernia, which is causing pain, or after overt trauma, and these conditions are generally not thought of as comprising an 'acute abdomen', because if the patient presents with tyre tracks across the abdomen, management may be fiendishly difficult but the diagnosis is blindingly obvious. The 'acute abdomen' (or acute abdominal pain) is therefore most often referred to in terms of the definition already given, and it is this definition which we shall follow in the subsequent sections of this chapter.

3. Common causes of acute abdominal pain

Inexperienced surgeons, and even most medical students, when asked for a list of causes of acute abdominal pain usually can recite a number of disease categories. However, in order to make a sensible decision, you need to know more than this, because the list of potential causes of acute abdominal pain is almost endless.

So as well as merely knowing the list of potential causes of acute abdominal pain, the surgeon, faced with a practical decision as to what to do about an individual patient, needs to know: (a) what are the *commonest* causes of pain to look for on the surgical wards in order that these may be considered first; and also (b) how the age and sex of the patient affects these overall values. In other words the surgeon needs the sort of information contained in Figure 5.2 and Table 5.1.

Appendicitis 25%
Diverticular disease 2%
Perforated ulcer 2%
Non-specific abdominal pain 45%
Cholecystitis 10%
Bowel obstruction 4%
Pancreatitis 2%
Renal colic 4%
Dyspepsia 5%

Figure 5.2 Common causes of acute abdominal pain on surgical wards, obtained from a multinational study of 15 000 patients. (From de Dombal F T (1988) *Scandinavian Journal of Gastroenterology*; **23** (suppl. 144): 35–42.

Table 5.1 Common causes of acute abdominal pain in particular age groups, obtained from a multinational study of 15 000 patients. (From de Dombal F T (1988) *Scandinavian Journal of Gastroenterology*; 23 (suppl. 144): 34–42.)

Age group	Common causes
Children	Intussusception Urinary-tract infection Hernia
Young adult males	Trauma Crohn's disease Alcohol
Young adult females	Urinary-tract infection Pelvic inflammatory disease Ovarian cyst Ectopic pregnancy Abortion

Figure 5.2 shows the results of a worldwide survey of over 15 000 cases of acute abdominal pain carried out under the auspices of the Research Committee of the World Organization of Gastroenterology, and summarizes the common surgical causes. Most of the categories will be familiar, but

one category, the commonest of all, may not be familiar, and is NSAP (non-specific abdominal pain). This category covers a myriad of causes of acute self-limiting pain where the patient recovers (sometimes after laparotomy) and goes home from hospital with no firm diagnosis being made.

You may argue that NSAP is therefore not a diagnosis at all and I would agree. It is however, in my own view, more honest to admit that the cause has not been established, and there is also a further and much more important justification for this term. The letters NSAP stand not only for *non-specific abdominal pain* but also for *non-surgical abdominal pain* (or as some American paramedics say, no-sweat abdominal pain!). Think back to the previous chapters. A diagnosis of NSAP may not indicate precisely what pathological process is going on, but it does indicate clearly how the situation is to be managed (e.g. without operation) and as such is a more helpful category than say mesenteric lymphadenitis. (How, incidentally, mesenteric lymphadenitis can be diagnosed without opening the abdomen, or even if the abdomen is opened, how one can be sure that the lymph nodes are the cause of the pain, has been a mystery to me for the last 25 years!)

Table 5.1 indicates some adjustments in thinking, which need to be made when dealing with specific age groups. For example, in dealing with children the surgeon needs to think about intussusception, urinary-tract infection and hernia, as these conditions are all relatively common. Indeed under the age of 30 months, intussusception is more commonly found than acute appendicitis. In the young adult male the effects of trauma and alcohol need to be considered, and Crohn's disease is an increasingly common cause in this age group. The young adult female, in addition to many of the conditions listed in Figure 5.2, may also suffer from urinary-tract infection, ovarian cyst, ectopic pregnancy, and particularly pelvic inflammatory disease (which accounts for approximately 5% of all presentations to hospital with acute abdominal pain in the United States, and is rapidly increasing in the UK as well). Finally, and just occasionally, a misdiagnosed abortion will cause the patient to present to the surgical wards.

I want to digress at this point and say a word or two about elderly patients. The elderly patient with acute abdominal pain presents a particularly difficult problem for 2 reasons. First, a wrong decision is much more likely to kill the patient. Mortality in the young adult from acute abdominal pain is around 0.1% overall, rising to 7% in those over 80. Second, the diagnostic accuracy in this age group is particularly low (only around 30% in many series). Studies have shown that this is frequently because the inexperienced surgeon never even considers the right diagnosis; or in other words, the inexperienced surgeon never considers the data in Table 5.1.

In particular 3 diagnostic categories tend to be missed, and all of these need to be considered by the prudent surgeon making an appropriate decision. First, studies have shown that 10% of patients over the age of 50 presenting to hospital with 'puzzling' acute abdominal pain have *cancer* as an underlying cause – usually large bowel cancer in Europe and North America and liver cancer in the Tropics. Second, 10% of patients in the over 70 years of age group with acute abdominal pain have a *vascular cause* (mesenteric insufficiency, aortic aneurysm, or myocardial infarction) underlying their condition. The situation regarding *perforation* is quite different in elderly patients. The appendix tends to perforate more quickly and more frequently in patients over the age of 50; and a number of studies have shown that elderly patients with generalized peritonitis are just as likely to have perforated their colon as perforated their appendix or a peptic ulcer.

Does this last point matter? Of course it does, not so much in diagnostic terms as in decision making terms. Remember, your job is not to tie a label on the patient but to decide what to do to sort out the patient's problem. It is all too easy for an inexperienced surgeon to open the abdomen through a grid-iron or upper right paramedian incision only to find a faeculent peritonitis and a perforated sigmoid colon to deal with. By now the patient may be extremely toxic. The inexperienced surgeon is out of his/her depth and appropriate help is not at hand. Small wonder that the mortality of this situation during and after operation is around 20% (even in the present day and age).

This is merely one example of the importance of knowing what you are dealing with, knowing the common causes and knowing the special circumstances that make particular diseases more likely. If you do not know what you are dealing with, it is unlikely that you will come up with the correct decision for the patient.

4. What information to acquire

We have already seen in previous pages the importance of collecting adequate and appropriate information from a patient both in terms of interview, examination, and special investigations. We have also seen that the process of learning the procedures tends to be confusing for the student and inexperienced surgeon, because each of their teachers tends to have his or her 'pet' list of symptoms or signs. The student is reluctant to question this information, but it does tend to become confusing when these various lists conflict with one another.

In the present context, the information form in Figure 5.3 may be of help. It is taken from a number of surveys and represents the consensus view of approximately 1000 surgeons worldwide who have (with their junior staff) used it to collect data for a number of surveys for the World Organization of Gastroenterology, WHO, the European Community, and the Department of Health in the UK. As such, it probably represents a reasonable starting point for the inexperienced surgeon or student, at least until experience is gained.

In looking at the figure, you may be perplexed by one of two problems. First, your own teacher's 'pet' symptom or sign may not be on the list. If so, this does not mean that your chief is wrong. It merely means that a consensus view from hundreds of surgeons around the world did not include this particular sign or symptom.

You may also have noticed that the abdominal pain chart used in these surveys does not include some of the informa-

Abdominal Pain Chart

NAME	REG NUMBER	
MALE/FEMALE AGE	FORM FILLED BY	
PRESENTATION (999. GP. etc)	DATE	TIME

PAIN

SITE

ONSET

PRESENT

RADIATION

AGGRAVATING FACTORS
movement
coughing
respiration
food
other
none

RELIEVING FACTORS
lying still
vomiting
antacides
food
other
none

PROGRESS
better
same
worse

DURATION

TYPE
intermittent
steady
colicky

SEVERITY
moderate
severe

HISTORY

NAUSEA
yes   no

VOMITING
yes   no

ANOREXIA
yes   no

PREV INDIGESTION
yes   no

JAUNDICE
yes   no

BOWELS
normal
constipation
diarrhoea
blood
mucus

MICTURITION
normal
frequency
dysuria
dark
haematuria

PREV SIMILAR PAIN
yes   no

PREV ABDO SURGERY
yes   no

DRUGS FOR ABDO PAIN
yes   no

♀ LMP

pregnant

Vag. discharge

dizzy/faint

EXAMINATION

MOOD
normal
distressed
anxious

SHOCKED
yes   no

COLOUR
normal
pale
flushed
jaundiced
cyanosed

TEMP   PULSE

BP

ABDO MOVEMENT
normal
poor nil
peristalsis

SCAR
yes   no

DISTENSION
yes   no

TENDERNESS

REBOUND
yes   no

GUARDING
yes   no

RIGIDITY
yes   no

MASS
yes   no

MURPHY'S
+ve   −ve

BOWEL SOUNDS
normal   absent   +++

RECTAL – VAGINAL TENDERNESS
left
right
general
mass
none

INITIAL DIAGNOSIS & PLAN

RESULTS
amylase
blood count (WBC)
computer
urine
X-ray
other

DIAG & PLAN AFTER INVEST

(time

DISCHARGE DIAGNOSIS

Figure 5.3 Data collection form for acute abdominal pain showing minimum dataset used in OMGE and EC multinational studies.

tion you need to make a decision. There is little about cardiovascular or chest problems, neurological problems, or past history which might influence you in deciding whether or not to operate on the patient. If this did cross your mind, you should modestly congratulate yourself, because it means that you are starting to think in terms of making decisions and not simply tying diagnostic labels on patients. Well done!

The information in the figure represents what is known as a 'minimum dataset'. It is by no means exclusive and you may well wish to add to it. It does however, represent a list of symptoms, signs and investigations considered prudent by surgeons worldwide; and as such, whilst you may wish to *add* to these symptoms and signs, you would be well advised not to *omit* any of them in your routine examination of the patient.

5. How to recognize common causes of pain

Once you know what acute abdominal pain is, know what conditions you are likely to encounter, and have secured adequate and appropriate data, you need to analyse the data so as to arrive at a sensible decision. We have already dealt with some aspects of this (is the patient telling the truth? has the patient really got acute abdominal pain or some other problem?) and we will assume that you are dealing with a genuine 'acute abdomen', and that the patient is not lying simply to avoid work or school.

In analysing the data, the first and most important point to remember is that you simply cannot analyse a 'full' case history all at once. As we discussed earlier (Chapter 3) and will consider further in Chapter 10, one day computers may perform this task routinely. Computers love data. You may have heard a computer complain of insufficient data, but you have never heard one complain that it has been given too much data! With humans however, in practice, the reverse is true. The human mind becomes easily overloaded. What you need therefore, in order to sort out patients with acute abdominal pain are 'short-lists' of symptoms helpful in the diagnosis of various common diseases.

This incidentally, is where your chief differs from you, for he/she has already developed by experience short-lists of critical symptoms for a variety of common diseases and problems. (Incidentally, once you have found out what these are, it is fascinating to watch an experienced surgeon at work because the questions that are asked will tell you the way in which the surgeon's mind is working if you listen carefully enough.)

We are faced here with a young lad suffering from possible appendicitis, and since you already know that a number of other diseases are unlikely, the problem you really have to sort out is whether or not acute appendicitis is present. On this judgement your decision about management will be made. What you therefore need is a short-list of symptoms and signs most helpful in distinguishing between acute appendicitis and non-specific or non-surgical abdominal pain. You need to distinguish, in other words, which of the features in Figure 5.3 you should pay particular attention to in making your judgement. This information is contained in Figure 5.4, which lists (on the basis of approximately 15 000 cases) the seven clinical features most likely to sort out the problem for you. Taken in isolation, none of them are pathognomonic; but in general terms the more of these features are present, the more likely the patient is to have acute appendicitis.

You will need to develop your own short-lists like this for each of the various conditions. Clearly there is insufficient space here to list them all, but since we mentioned cancer in the elderly patient it may be appropriate to add a couple of further lists, Figure 5.5, as an example of the sort of 'short-list' you will need to develop from your own experience.

Pain moving to right lower quadrant
Aggravated by movement, cough
Nausea, vomiting and anorexia
Flushing (normal body temperature)
Focal tenderness, right lower quadrant
Rebound and guarding
Tender on right side per rectum

Figure 5.4 Seven features most likely to predict acute appendicitis at interview and examination of a patient with acute abdominal pain. The more of these present, the more likely the patient has acute appendicitis.

> Over 60 years of age
> Pain over 48 h
> Pain getting worse
> Recent change in bowel habit
> Dysuria, increased frequency
> Abdominal distension
> Abdominal mass.

Figure 5.5 Same analysis as Figure 5.4, but for elderly patients with cancer masquerading as acute abdominal pain. Never send away a puzzling elderly patient without ensuring that someone will follow-up the case.

6. How to make an appropriate decision

You know what you are dealing with. You have acquired appropriate and adequate information by careful interview, careful physical examination, and possibly investigation of the patient. You know for example, how many of the features indicating acute appendicitis are present in this individual patient. It is now time to make a decision.

As we saw in an earlier chapter, there is a world of difference between tying a diagnostic label on the patient and making a decision in order to manage the situation and solve the patient's problem. I hope you will also remember from an earlier chapter that the first step in decision making is to outline the possible options and the critical decisions that need to be made in order to deal with the problem. In this case there are four decisions:

1. Should the patient be admitted to hospital?
2. To which service should the patient be admitted?
3. Should the patient be operated upon?
4. Is any other management necessary?

If these points crossed your mind before reading them, again congratulate yourself, because you are beginning to think like a surgeon and not like a medical student. If you considered turning back to Figure 5.4 to help you in making the decision, even better, because it indicates you understand the need to take sensible decisions using appropriate evidence.

Over the years I have tended to use the data in Figure 5.4 as a simple 'rule of thumb' for dealing with suspected appendicitis, as follows:

- if a patient has none of those features, or possibly one, all things being equal the patient can be allowed home
- if a patient has two of the features (any two) there is possibly little need to admit or operate on a patient immediately, but a spell on the observation ward may be appropriate
- if a patient has three (any three) they probably should be admitted to the surgical wards and observed
- if a patient who has four of these features (any four) the patient should (all things being equal) be considered very seriously for operation.

Over the years I have also made a series of friendly wagers with my students. If a medical student can show me a patient with four or more of the features in Figure 5.4, who does not have a surgical abdomen (e.g. acute appendicitis), I award them half a pint of beer at the end of the 2-month period. Conversely, to any student who can show me a patient with genuine appendicitis, and who does *also* not have at *least* two of the features, goes a full pint of beer.

I generally pay out about half a pint every 2 months. You will notice that I am not making a similar offer to all readers of this book. But when you compare one error (on the side of caution) per 2 months, with the current overall diagnostic accuracy around the UK (and elsewhere) of 45%, you may feel that the approach we have just discussed, and also list of features in Figure 5.4 has something to offer in routine clinical practice.

6

The decision to operate

The decision of whether or not to operate on a particular patient is central to all surgical decision making, and as such requires detailed consideration. Not surprisingly, it is a decision that many inexperienced surgeons often find to be extremely difficult (as indeed do some of their most experienced colleagues on occasion).

Part of the problem results from the fact that, perhaps surprisingly, many medical students and inexperienced surgeons have never really thought about the decision to operate in any structured or analytical way until the decision is forced upon them. It is not their fault! Medical students are understandably reluctant to query a senior colleague's decision to operate (or not to operate) and, to be brutally frank, their textbooks do little to help them. Often, the decision to operate, which is arguably the most difficult decision a surgeon has to make, is glossed over in a single line; for example, 'the treatment of acute appendicitis is immediate surgery'.

Like most dogmatic statements, this one is generally true, but not invariably. With increasing experience, the young surgeon comes to realize that there are two problems attached to this simplistic statement. First of all, one can never be absolutely certain before operation that the patient does have acute appendicitis; and, secondly, there are some situations (extreme high-risk patients, remote situations, lack of adequate facilities for surgery, and patients with long-standing pain and an appendix mass) where the decision best suited to that particular patient's interests may well be to withhold immediate operation.

Moreover, many patients with disease that may or may not warrant surgery present a far more difficult problem to the surgeon as regards the decision whether or not to operate (e.g. the elderly, frail patient with partial intestinal obstruction, the 45-year-old bus driver with H_2 blocker-resistant peptic ulcer, the frightened young girl with severe acute inflammatory bowel disease). The list is endless and provides much anxiety and soul-searching, on occasion even for the most experienced surgeon.

To watch a master craftsman weighing up the evidence and making up his or her mind and arriving at a decision whether or not to operate on a particular patient, is one of the most rewarding experiences for a student or inexperienced doctor. Or rather, it should be, but often it is not. Often surgeons, like other doctors, are notoriously bad at explaining their train of thought and the inexperienced doctor or student simply does not have sufficient information or knowledge about the decision to operate to follow the process that is going on. This is a double disaster, because apart from missing out on the educational experience, the student also misses out on the fun.

So in this chapter we are going to look at a decision to operate, and we are going to do so in a structured way, imagining (as is usual in this book) that we are faced with a patient who may or may not warrant surgery, that no one else is around or available to make the decision or help with the decision, but that a decision must be made in the interests of the patient. This is the challenge. How should we proceed?

The three basic questions

When faced with a patient (any patient) in this situation, there are many considerations that spring to mind. What has been the response to conservative therapy? What about the patient as a person? What type of surgery would be best? It is not surprising that students and inexperienced surgeons become confused. So in order to understand the decision making process further, and in the interests of clarity, we shall consider here three basic questions that need to be answered in each and every case before the decision to

proceed with surgery is taken. These questions are as
follows:

1. **Can surgery offer anything for this particular condition?**
2. **Does this particular patient have an indication for surgery?**
3. **In this individual patient, do the likely potential benefits of
   surgery outweigh the risks of performing the operation?**

These 3 questions form a natural and logical sequence. If
the answer to any of them is negative, then there is no point
whatsoever in proceeding further. Only if the answer to all
three questions is affirmative should the decision to operate
be taken.

I very strongly recommend that every time you see a
particular patient you should ask yourself these three questions – preferably before anyone else has seen the patient or
made a decision – and then watch what happens as the
eventual decision is made. So let us look at each of these in
turn.

1. Does surgery have anything to offer?

The first step in the decision to operate is clearly to decide
whether for the patient's condition there is a surgical treatment that has anything to offer. Often this decision is very
clear-cut, and there are a large number of conditions for
which surgery has absolutely nothing whatsoever to offer.
Under these circumstances the decision has already been
made and there is no point in proceeding further. Equally,
there are some conditions for which the standard management under normal circumstances clearly involves surgery,
such as acute appendicitis.

However, there are a number of situations in clinical
medicine where it is not absolutely clear whether surgery has
anything to offer for the particular condition from which the
patient suffers. In these circumstances it may be helpful in
deciding whether to operate, to consider what surgical
treatment actually has to offer for the disease in question.

This is best done by reviewing the potential benefits of surgery, which are listed below, in order to determine whether one or more of these benefits is likely to be obtained in the patient's particular circumstances, and thereby determine what exactly you are trying to achieve for a particular patient.

Maintain life
Prolong life
Relieve or abolish pain
Improve or restore function
Improve the quality of life

The potential benefits of surgery

A good deal of surgery is performed with the aim of *maintaining or prolonging the patient's life*. An obvious example of the former concerns the patient with acute abdominal pain in whom a diagnosis of acute appendicitis or perforated peptic ulcer has been made. Here the aim of surgery is clearly to maintain the patient's life, because without surgery the patient has an increased risk of dying. Equally, much cancer surgery is performed with the aim of prolonging the patient's life, because without surgery there is very good evidence that the patient's life expectancy will be drastically shortened.

The second important aim of surgery, in patients whose life is not threatened by their disease, is the *relief (partial or total) of pain*. Again examples are numerous, such as the patient with duodenal ulcer who is suffering from severe episodes of pain, which has not been alleviated, or the ulcer healed, by standard forms of medical therapy.

There are however, a number of areas of surgery where the aim is neither to maintain or prolong life, nor to relieve or abolish pain, but to *improve the function* of the part of the body in question. Under this heading comes a great deal of orthopaedic surgery, which not only is performed to relieve or abolish pain, but is also performed on many occasions to improve function, ranging from hip replacements to operations on nerves and tendons in the limbs.

Finally, and shading into the above aim, comes the aim of *improving the quality of life* of the patient. Often surgery may be performed solely or partly with this aim in mind. Examples range from the orthopaedic operations just discussed to many forms of plastic surgery, which only rarely maintain or prolong the patient's life (or abolish pain), but which may be extremely important in improving the quality of life of the particular patient.

Some surgeons even start at the outset by constructing, with the patient's cooperation, a list of goals, which the treatment is designed to achieve. I am not sure I would go as far as this, but it is extremely helpful to make sure that both surgeon and patient at the outset understand very clearly what is intended to be achieved by the treatment.

Summary – the first step

So the first step in decision making is to decide whether surgery has anything to offer. If on the one hand it is clear that there is no reason to expect any of the benefits listed above from surgical management, then clearly one need proceed no further. The decision not to operate has already been made in this instance. If on the other hand surgery does have something to offer, then one can proceed to the next step in decision making, and this is to decide whether in the particular patient's case there is a specific indication for surgical treatment, and to decide what that indication is.

2. Indications for surgery

I am constantly saddened by the responses of students or inexperienced surgeons when asked to list the indications for surgery in a particular disease. Often, they stumble through one or two indications that they have managed to remember from a long list in a textbook, but it is quite clear they have not thought about this in any logical or sensible way.

It is not surprising that this should be so, and once again it is hardly their fault, because there are innumerable diseases and each disease has its own particular indications, and it is virtually impossible to remember them all at once. So clearly some kind of framework is needed in order to decide whether a particular indication for sugery exists in a specific patient. This is set out in summary in Table 6.1 and we shall now discuss these various aspects in turn.

Table 6.1 The indications for surgery

Type of sugery	Indications
Emergency surgery	Disease threatens life Complications threaten life (bleeding, blocking, bursting)
Urgent surgery	Failure of conservative management to control severe attack of disease
Effective surgery	Chronic symptoms Cancer (proven or suspected) Complications Cosmetics
Prophylactic surgery	Prevention of future problems (e.g. cancer development)

Types of surgery

The inexperienced student often thinks of 'surgery' as a single entity. This is wrong. Surgical procedures range from the heroic (with high mortality risk) to minimal (low risk) procedures, such as laser coagulation, or some of the new 'minimally invasive' procedures coming into routine use.

Also, surgery takes many forms (emergency, elective, prophylactic and so on). Therefore, in working out whether an indication for surgery exists in a particular patient, it is extremely helpful to consider the various types of surgery separately, because each type of surgery has a specific set of indications. It is helpful to work through the types of surgery in Table 6.1, and rather than considering whether surgery *per se* is indicated, consider in turn whether emergency surgery (or elective surgery) is indicated in a particular patient. This we shall now do, and the benefits of working through the types of surgery in this structured way will become clear as we proceed.

Emergency surgery

Emergency surgery is probably best defined as surgery that will not wait for the next surgical list. As well as the obvious implications as regards time, there are organizational implications. Often a decision to proceed to emergency surgery involves a decision to operate in a specific theatre designated for this purpose with all that implies – making the theatre ready, arranging for different staff to be present, and so on. So emergency surgery clearly needs to be separated from all other forms of surgery; and indeed the indications for surgery in this situation are quite different from the indications for other types of surgery.

Emergency surgery is performed by and large when *in the immediate future either the disease threatens life, or the complications of the disease threaten life.* Two excellent examples of this are those we considered earlier. Acute appendicitis clearly threatens life and therefore warrants emergency surgery. Duodenal ulcer does not necessarily threaten life but a perforated duodenal ulcer does; hence perforation of a duodenal ulcer warrants emergency surgery, not because the disease itself threatens life, but because this added complication does.

The complications that threaten life are of course many, and the main ones are listed in Table 6.1. It may be an aid to memory to remember that in colloquial language these all begin with the letter B: *blocking* (e.g. obstruction of the bowel or an artery), *bursting* (e.g. perforation of a viscus such as duodenum, appendix or colon) and *bleeding* (e.g. severe haemorrhage from any site) are the main indications for emergency surgery and taken together account for the vast majority of operations performed under this heading.

Therefore, in deciding whether there is an indication for surgery in a particular patient, first of all consider whether an emergency operation is necessary, and look for the three main indications listed in Table 6.1. If these are present, then there is an indication for emergency surgery. If they are not, less dramatic measures may still be indicated.

Urgent surgery

The second type of operation, urgent surgery, differs from the emergency situation in that there is judged to be time to wait until the next operating list and no need to involve an emergency procedure. Usually, a few days are involved; but only rarely is urgent surgery delayed longer than this, and rarely for more than about a week. There is really one overriding indication for urgent surgery: *failure of the patient to respond to conservative forms of therapy in a severe attack of disease.*

There is a very important principle here, and that is the *integration* of conservative and operative treatment. In planning your management (e.g. in dealing with a patient with severe inflammatory bowel disease), it is important to have an integrated plan *from the outset.* Thus a patient with a severe attack of ulcerative colitis may well be given an intensive regime involving steroids and sulphasalazine (or one of the newer 5–ASA derivatives); but it is in the best interests of the patient if everyone concerned is quite clear that if over a period of a few days this regime does not improve the symptoms then urgent surgery will be amply warranted.

In the case of inflammatory bowel disease (and in particular ulcerative colitis), over 200 British gastroenterologists were surveyed. The majority would set this particular time period (of careful observation) at between 5 and 9 days. I personally feel there is rather good evidence (see p. 133) for the shorter (5 day) period but the precise time is immaterial to the discussion here. What matters is the clear understanding by both patient and doctor from the outset that failure to respond within an agreed time period to conservative treatment is an indication for urgent surgery to be considered. Time and again, studies have shown that if this integrated approach is not pursued there is an understandable but erroneous tendency to let matters drift for day after day in the hope of improvement; and time and again this delay has been shown to result in an increased mortality for the patient.

Elective surgery
The vast majority of operations performed in most industrialized countries are performed electively. It is well that this should be so because surgery is always safer if time can be

afforded to prepare the patient thoroughly and appropriately for the operation in question.

Before dealing further with the indications for elective surgery, we need to be clear what we mean by the word 'elective'. Of course, the word does not mean (as some students imagine) that one elects whether or not to operate; elective surgery merely implies that one can choose the *time* of operation. Even this is not an absolute rule because obviously the patient with a suspicious breast lump warrants surgery earlier than a patient with long-standing and relatively minor varicose veins. Nevertheless, in all elective surgery, there is some lattitude as to the precise timing of the operation. The indications for elective surgery are completely different from those concerning more urgent situations.

Again for ease of memory, it may be helpful to recall that the major indications for elective surgery all begin with the letter C. The first and most common indication is *chronic symptoms*. Indeed, this is probably the commonest indication for surgery and it is not difficult to think of examples. The patient with a painful arthritic hip, the patient with third degree haemorrhoids, and the patient with duodenal ulcer whose pain does not respond to antacids or H_2 blockers, all suffer from chronic symptoms. It is this chronicity of their symptoms (despite the best efforts of conservative therapy), which forms the indication for elective surgery.

The next most frequent indication for elective surgery is *cancer, either proven or suspected*. It is not difficult to cite a gastric cancer proven by endoscopic biopsy as an indication for surgery; but it is equally important to realize that in many instances the indication for surgery may not be proven but merely suspected cancer (e.g. a suspicious breast lump, a darkening, enlarging, and bleeding lesion in the skin, or a stricture in the colon seen on barium enema). In each instance the patient may be relatively free from pain or other symptoms and it is the suspicion of cancer (even after non-operative investigation such as barium enema or endoscopic biopsy), which forms the indication for sugery.

The next group of indications for elective surgery concerns *complications* of a particular disease. Again, thinking of inflammatory bowel disease, the disease in the bowel may be quiescent, but the patient may suffer from a troublesome perianal complication such as abscess, fistula or fissure. In this instance it is the complication of the disease rather than the disease itself that requires surgery, usually of an elective type.

The final indication for elective surgery, which accounts for a significantly increasing number of operations, is a *cosmetic* problem. Of course in some parts of the world cosmetic surgery is a major industry in its own right, but there are often situations in routine clinical practice when the cosmetic effect of a lesion must be taken into account when assessing the situation. Examples again are numerous: the unsightly skin lesion, the large swelling in the neck from a benign thyroid lesion, and even on occasion prominent and unsightly varicose veins (though the wearing of tights seems to have reduced this aspect of cosmetic surgery).

Prophylactic surgery

If the patient has none of the indications we have discussed so far, and is relatively symptom-free, then prophylactic surgery may still be indicated. Often the basis for prophylactic surgery is the known risk to the patient of cancer development at some time in the future. However, this consideration does not apply to cancer alone, but to any severe complication; prophylactic surgery may be indicated to head off trouble in the future in a variety of diseases.

For example, consider the global traveller who perforates a (hitherto unsuspected) peptic ulcer while in foreign parts, and returns home having undergone simple suture of the perforation. The patient may be relatively symptom-free, and in ordinary circumstances no further surgical treatment may be warranted. However, if the patient announces his or her intention to travel again to parts of the world where surgery may not be available, then operation may be indicated purely on a prophylactic basis, not on the grounds of the present situation, but to head off a repeat performance in the future.

Speaking of foreign parts incidentally, and thinking of the value of prophylactic surgery, you might reflect upon the *high* incidence of strangulation in groin hernia in the tropics and the *low* incidence in the western world, following widespread (prophylactic) repair of uncomplicated hernias. Prophylactic surgery at its best.

Summary – the second step
The second step in assessing a patient for surgery, and in deciding whether or not to operate, is to review the list of potential indications for surgery. If the patient has none of the indications we have considered, then it is rather unlikely that surgery will be indicated. If on the other hand, one (or possibly more) of the indications we have listed are present in a particular patient, then the patient has a disease that responds to surgery, and has an indication for surgery. Surgery may well be indicated in this case. However, before deciding that surgery should be performed, there is another important consideration to think about, and this final consideration we shall now discuss.

3. Risks and benefits

The third vital question that we need to ask ourselves in dealing with a patient (i) who has a disease for which surgery can offer some benefit, and (ii) who has a clear-cut indication for surgery, is a simple one: in this particular patient do the prospective benefits of surgery outweigh the additional risks to the patient of the operation in question?

In recent years a whole scientific discipline, in many walks of life, has evolved around the subject of what has become known as 'risk-benefit analysis'; because much of this argument has involved mathematicians and statisticians, it has only a minor place in this particular book, although some helpful references for the interested reader are appended at the end. For now, however, it follows that in order to make an appropriate judgement about a particular patient, we need to have clear information on a series of topics, namely:

- the risk of operating on a patient
- the likelihood of benefit from the operation in question.

We also need to know, in order to arrive at a balanced assessment, answers to further questions, namely:

- the likelihood of benefit from continued conservative therapy
- the potential risk to the patient of continued conservative therapy.

Some simple examples
In this situation I personally find it helpful to view the whole subject of risk-benefit analysis in the form of a set of scales or balances, which may tip in favour of surgery or conservative therapy depending upon the situation in question.

A couple of simple examples are shown in Figure 6.1a and 6.1b. Figure 6.1a concerns a patient with classical symptoms and signs of acute appendicitis. In this situation we know that the risk of surgery is 0.1% in terms of mortality (providing the appendix has not yet perforated) with a 10–20% morbidity following operation, usually of a relatively minor nature. We know also that the disease will be completely cured if the operation is successful. By contrast we know that conservative management has little to offer, that the chance of perforation, if untreated, is 25–30%, and we know that the mortality is increased by a factor of 10 if the patient perforates. Under these circumstances surgery is clearly warranted.

By contrast (Figure 6.1b), in the patient with distal ulcerative colitis and little in the way of symptoms, we know that, while surgery will eradicate the disease, the mortality of proctocolectomy is at least 1–2%, with a morbidity of 30–40%, and with the attendant disadvantages to the patient of a permanent ileostomy. We also know that conservative treatment in the form of maintenance sulphasalazine has a very good chance of maintaining the patient in remission, and we further know that there are relatively few risks of major complications in association with distal ulcerative colitis. Under these circumstances surgery is clearly not indicated, and the balance in this particular patient tips towards continued conservative management.

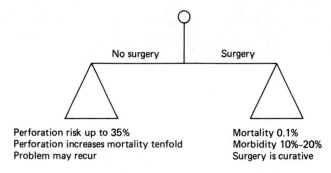

Perforation risk up to 35%
Perforation increases mortality tenfold
Problem may recur

Mortality 0.1%
Morbidity 10%-20%
Surgery is curative

Clearly in this situation the balance tilts in favour of surgery

Figure 6.1a Risk-benefit analysis for a patient with 'classical' appendicitis.

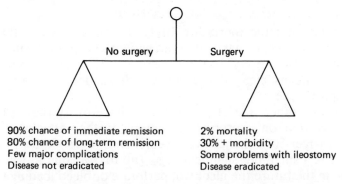

90% chance of immediate remission
80% chance of long-term remission
Few major complications
Disease not eradicated

2% mortality
30% + morbidity
Some problems with ileostomy
Disease eradicated

In these circumstances, despite the fact that surgery eradicates the disease
the balance tips in favour of continued conservative care

Figure 6.1b Risk-benefit analysis for a patient with distal, mild ulcerative colitis.

More difficult problems

In some situations the scales may be very finely balanced
indeed. Consider Figure 6.2, which deals with a 50-year-old
bus driver suffering from duodenal ulcer, who suffers inter-
mittently from pain associated with a duodenal ulcer, and
where his pain is only partly relieved by conservative
therapy. Here the decision may be very difficult. On one
side of the scales we know the mortality of operation is less

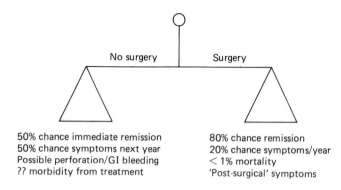

Figure 6.2 Same analysis as Figure 6.1a and 6.1b, showing risk and benefits in patients where the 'pros and cons' of surgical treatment are finely balanced. This is where 'professional judgement' plays a part (see text).

than 1% and the morbidity 10–15%. We also know that there is a 70–80% chance that the patient's symptoms will be improved by surgery. But this is not a 100% chance, so it is by no means clear that surgery will render the patient symptom-free.

On the other side of the scales we have every reason to suspect that on conservative therapy further attacks will occur (over 50% chance every year), and we also know that there is a small but significant risk (up to 5%) that at some time in the future the ulcer will perforate or bleed leading to significantly enhanced risk to life. The scales are finely balanced: so what do we do?

This case demonstrates some of the limitations of formal 'decision analysis' (p. 53) and illustrates why 'professional judgement' is so important. Here, where the scales are finely balanced, we are in what our American colleagues describe as the 'Close Call Zone'. Technically it would be possible to perform the sort of decision analysis shown on p. 53 and arrive at an answer – 'operate' or 'do not operate'. To do so however, we have to make assumptions about the patient's preferences and choices, assumptions that are, on the whole, correctly and speedily made by an experienced surgeon after discussion with the patient, but which are frightfully difficult to put into precise mathematical terms.

So, under these circumstances, is operation warranted? Clearly the patient has a disease that responds to surgery, and clearly there is an indication (chronic symptoms), for elective surgery. But in this particular patient it is a matter of judgement as to whether the symptoms are sufficiently severe to warrant surgery, or whether one should persist with further conservative management.

This then is where 'professional judgement' comes in. We discuss 'professional judgement' in more detail elsewhere. The point I am making in this chapter is that it is impossible to make an objective and appropriate judgement unless one clearly understands both the risks and the benefits of continued conservative management and operative intervention. Indeed, unless one clearly understands both the risks and the benefits of the alternative forms of therapy, it is misleading, and arguably highly unethical, to hide behind the cloak of 'clinical judgement' and (worse) 'clinical freedom' in making a snap judgement and an arbitrary decision.

Note, finally, that we have glossed over another important problem – we have assumed you know what the diagnosis is, and that may not always be the case. Consider for a moment the patient with suspected appendicitis. If you are sure appendicitis is present, the decision to operate is usually obvious; similarly if you are sure appendicitis is *not* present, the decision not to operate is equally obvious. But can you ever be completely sure, and what do you do if you are *not* sure? At what level of suspicion do you decide to proceed to surgery? Here decision analysis can become quite useful; and since the principles are the same for *all* surgical decisions, they are dealt with in another chapter (see p. 53).

For now however, remember that you cannot sensibly decide whether or not to operate unless you know the likely risks and benefits to the patient, both of surgical and conservative management. Make sure that by the time you come to make the decision you have learnt what these risks and benefits are, and you will have taken an important step towards making sensible decisions most likely to benefit your patients.

So to sum up, each and every decision for or against operative intervention should be made on simple grounds, by considering the answers to the three questions we have discussed earlier in this chapter – can surgery offer anything? is there an indication for surgery? and 'in this patient' do the prospective benefits of surgery outweigh the risks of performing the operation? The questions are indeed simple; the problem is that sometimes the answers are extremely complex. Patients are people, and (*pace* the decision analysts) sometimes decisions are made not on mathematical grounds or purely logical grounds, but on grounds of humanity, because both surgeons and patients are human beings. Thus, while the objective situation may be quite clear-cut, ethical considerations and the management of the patient as a person may raise considerable difficulties; and it is these difficulties that we shall discuss in a subsequent chapter.

7

Post-operative decisions

In an ideal world a separate chapter on post-operative decision making would have no place in a small text such as this. In days gone by, the post-operative management of patients consisted of little more than pain relief. Nowadays the subject has become so complex that to deal fully with it would require a whole book in itself. Indeed one of the finest surgical textbooks ever written, by Professor Francis D. Moore from Harvard University, devotes approximately 1000 pages to precisely this topic.

Unfortunately, however the world is not ideal. Much as we might like to be able to do so, very few of us are capable of thinking in complex scientific terms when awakened at 3 a.m. after 30 minutes sleep. In fact, if one takes a straw poll amongst newly qualified doctors (and I have taken many!) it is this aspect of their work that causes them most concern of all – not because the average problem is complex in itself, but because they find themselves alone on the wards and unable to contact senior colleagues for support without picking up the telephone and disturbing *their* sleep. To complicate the issue further, this aspect of clinical care is poorly taught (or often not taught at all). Therefore it is almost impossible to pick up what to do by 'osmosis', without spending many hours as a student sitting around on the wards at night and waiting for something to happen. I have not in my experience met many students who do this; and hence some newly qualified surgeons find that they have not considered the problems of immediate post-operative management until their first night on duty.

So, the purpose of this chapter is not to deal in detail with complex situations or decisions, but to offer some brief guidelines on the general way to proceed, which may be of some assistance until personal experience has been built up. Note that in doing so, the chapter will concentrate upon the immediate post-operative situation, although the principles apply to most similar situations that occur throughout clinical care. As in previous chapters, we shall concentrate upon a specific patient to illustrate a more general method of approach. The problem to be discussed in this chapter is encapsulated as follows:

You are on duty on the surgical wards of a large general surgical unit. It is Friday night, everyone else has gone home and you are responsible not only for your patients but those of a colleague who has left for the weekend. You retire to bed at 3 a.m. Fifteen minutes later the phone rings. The ward staff ask you to have a look at a 55-year-old man who underwent synchronous combined abdomino-perineal resection of the rectum 2 days previously. The message you receive is vague ("he doesn't look very well") and because the patient is normally being cared for by your colleague's firm, you know very little about him. You are on your own. No one else is in the hospital. How do you proceed?

Of course, I fully realize this is to simplify the situation. The patient's problem may be due to almost anything, and you may be faced with a very complex situation. At 3 a.m. however, after virtually no sleep, the biggest danger is not that you will face a rare, complex irremediable problem, but that you will miss something simple and treatable. Most young surgeons (if they are being honest) admit to considerable worry in this situation. So here are some suggestions, which, although not complete in themselves, may help you sort out the patient's problem.

Rule 1. You must attend
Throughout clinical medicine, this is an important and general principle. Until you personally assess the patient, you really have no idea what the problem actually is, whatever the message you may have received, and it is of course quite impossible to defend subsequent action or

lawsuit if you have failed to attend a patient. There is however a particular difficulty here. Often the message you will receive in these circumstances is extremely vague – for example "Mr. X doesn't look very well", or something similarly vague. Nevertheless, you must attend.

Incidentally, if you want to avoid being called with such a vague message, you may care to follow my own practice in this situation. Before retiring to bed, go round all the problem patients under your care for the night and in case of any doubt or worry leave specific instructions (e.g. call me if the pulse rises above 100, or the blood pressure falls below 120 systolic). Even if you do not do this, you should remember that experienced nurses often develop a 'sixth sense', which (though it may not be based on modern biochemistry or physiology) is often uncannily accurate in predicting the development of problems in a patient at 3 a.m. in the morning.

So, the first rule is that whatever the message you must attend. Those of you who have read the relevant books, or have watched the movie or television series, *All Creatures Great and Small*, may recall that the experienced veterinary surgeon Seigfried Farnon said much the same thing to the young James Herriot. If this rule is good enough for the management of farm animals in the Dales of Yorkshire, then it is certainly good enough for your patients! You must attend.

Rule 2. Identify the type of problem
When you arrive on the wards the first thing to do is to assess the situation, and make up your mind as rapidly as possible as to what sort of situation and problem you are dealing with. You will, of course already know about the 10–20s check (a quick look at the patient's respiration, temperature, pulse, consciousness level, and so on). While you are performing this check, it is helpful at this time to classify the patient's problem under one of four or five headings in your own mind. It is particularly helpful to do this right at the outset, because the categories are all treated differently. The categories broadly speaking are as follows:

- no problem
- minor problem
- serious problem
- dead +/−
- irretrievable.

At the top end of the scale, sometimes the problem will be over by the time you get there. The patient will appear to be perfectly well and may even be resentful of having been awoken. It is however, important to remember that this does not imply that there never was a problem. The wise young resident surgeon keeps his/her cool, thanks the nursing staff politely and returns to bed. In doing so, however, you should always make a point of insisting upon being rung again if things get worse or recur. Ideally, you should (as discussed earlier) specify what your 'cut-off points' are (e.g. if the systolic blood pressure falls below 120 again call me). You should remember that the nursing staff who called you (even for 'nothing') were well intentioned and apprehensive, and just occasionally you will be extremely glad you did not get angry at being called 'unnecessarily' when you get called back half an hour later to see the 'non-problem' or 'minor problem' that is by now a full blown crisis.

At the other end of the scale, you may be confused by the concept 'dead +/−'. The rationale for this category, however, is very simple, because it relates to management. Patients who are on the point of death, or patients who have just died as you arrive on the ward are equally both candidates for cardiopulmonary resuscitation. You should of course be thoroughly familiar with these procedures, and it is not the purpose of this book to deal with this in detail. However, a few pointers may be helpful.

First, on moving into a new unit or a new hospital, it is an absolute priority to identify for yourself the procedures to be followed in making a 'crash call'. I personally arrived (by chance) on the wards to find a distraught young surgeon trying to summon the resuscitation team by dialling 999, but the code number in the hospital in question was not 999 but 222. Second, in this connection, it is a priority to identify beforehand any candidates who are not to be resuscitated.

Do not under any circumstances allow yourself to be faced with this decision at 3 a.m. in the morning if you can help it. (Of course if no such information exists or if you are unsure, the only safe thing to do is to exert maximum resuscitation efforts and worry about it later.)

Finally, you do rather tend to look silly if you call out the cardiopulmonary resuscitation team in an attempt to resuscitate a patient who has been dead for some hours. You should remember that the nursing staff only see the average post-operative patient a few times each night, and most of us who have been around the wards for some time have experienced an emergency call to a patient who has been dead for some hours. Make sure, therefore, if your assessment indicates that the patient is no longer living, that you check quickly for the signs of irretrievability, such as rigor mortis or post-mortem lividity, which may help you avoid an embarrassing error.

Rule 3. The 'serious' problem – take it system by system

The patients who will give you the most trouble, however, are in the middle group. These patients obviously have a serious problem, but the problem is not clear from your initial brief 20s assessment. Unless you follow some overall scheme, you will eventually finish up sooner or later missing the patient's problem completely.

Sometimes the problem is obvious, and you can proceed with management. Often you will be faced with an ill patient but no obvious cause, and of course the difficulty is that the *potential* causes for the patient's condition are endless. By far the easiest way to deal with the situation is to tackle the problems system by system – looking first for the commonest causes of post-operative illness. In the next section of this chapter we shall proceed in this fashion, and look at some of the common problems and some pitfalls in recognizing them.

Surgical problems

If you are faced with a patient who is unwell following operation, the most common underlying cause of the situation is that something related to the operation has gone wrong. There are three problems in particular that should cross your mind at this stage, before any other problems are considered. These are:

- bleeding
- dehiscence
- infection.

Each of these developments may be blindingly obvious and you may have no difficulty in recognizing the situation. However, this is by no means always the case. So, as a priority, you will need to inspect both the wound itself and the area around it looking for bleeding, dehiscence, or infection. Remember that in abdominal surgery, dehiscence may not merely relate to the wound but to the dehiscence of an anastomosis that has broken down within the abdominal cavity. You will need to remember that in abdominal surgery any of these conditions may present without focal or overt signs but merely as a developing generalized perito- nitis. It is good practice at this point to remove the wound dressing and inspect the wound thoroughly, and in this particular patient's case you should remember that the patient has more than one wound and inspect the perineal wound as well. It is always embarrassing when a senior colleague, whom you have called in to see your 'puzzling' patient, demonstrates within 20s that the patient is lying in a pool of blood, which you have not detected by failing to inspect the perineal wound.

Cardiovascular problems
Assuming that the wound is intact, the abdomen is soft, and there is no obvious evidence of bleeding, and you are satisfied that problems related to the operation have not occurred, the next most common set of problems relate to the cardiovascular system. There are once again three problems that occur more often than the others. These are:

- myocardial infarction
- heart failure
- cerebrovascular accident.

Of course you know perfectly well how to recognize these conditions, but in the post-operative patient there are some special situations, and one or two extra pointers may be of help. First of all, in surgical patients, *beware the silent infarct*. The post-operative patient may complain of typical chest pain and in this situation the diagnosis may be obvious. However, many a patient with post-operative myocardial infarction has *already recently been given a substantial dose of analgesics for post-operative pain* (and this particularly applies early in the night when patients tend to be given analgesics by the nursing staff to help them to sleep). Thus the typical chest pain, which is so helpful in making the diagnosis, may be absent or slight.

Next, as regards heart failure, you will of course be well aware of the classical features of both left- and right-sided cardiac failure and well able to make a diagnosis in a clear cut case. Remember however, one further important point as regards left-sided failure. A few moments may well have elapsed between the call for your help and your arrival at the patient's bedside. The classical breathlessness may therefore not be present at the time you see the patient, because by that time the patient may be sitting up, and the breathlessness that caused distress (when supine) has decreased. If this has happened, you can usually gain some clue to the situation by listening carefully to the bases of both lungs. If you detect bilateral fine crepitations, suspect left-sided heart failure, and react accordingly.

Finally, in relation to cerebrovascular accident, if you should find some transient evidence of neurological abnormality, remember that some patients, particularly the elderly, react to post-operative analgesia by dropping their blood pressure quite markedly. In these circumstances, you should certainly think very carefully before further analgesia is administered.

Respiratory problems
If you get as far as this, and are still unsure at this stage of your examination of the cause of the patient's problem, the next system to think about is the respiratory system. As before, there are many problems that may occur. But in

general terms there are three conditions that commonly cause difficulty after operation. These are:

- lobular atelectasia
- chest infection
- pulmonary embolism.

They are listed in this order because this is the rough chronological order in which you will encounter them. Thus, whilst pulmonary embolism is not unknown in the first few hours post-operatively, it is more commonly encountered a few days afterwards. Similarly, lobular atelectasia is more commonly encountered in the first hours after operation (rather than several days later).

Once again, a few comments and pointers may be helpful. In the first day or two post-operatively the commonest respiratory problem is lobular atelectasia. This is particularly likely to occur when the secretions in the tracheobronchial tree are somewhat viscid, and/or the patient is reluctant to cough because it is painful. You may diagnose this by listening to the chest (widespread scattered rhonchi) but sometimes it can also be diagnosed from the chart. Indeed, what is known as the 'triple spike' (elevation of temperature, pulse and respiration all at once) should alert you to the possibility of lobular atalectasia even before you examine the patient. Remember that in the first day or two, this condition is more likely than chest infection, and as well as antibiotics you will need to consider physiotherapy, which may on occasion be life-saving.

Finally, a word or two concerning pulmonary embolism may be helpful. You may have been taught to look for this by seeking calf-vein tenderness or even Homan's sign (pain in the calf on dorsiflection of the foot). You should remember, however, that all that often it is not the calf veins that produce fatal pulmonary emboli. The fatal pulmonary emboli usually come from more proximal veins in the pelvis, particularly after surgery in that area. If you find unilateral chest signs, rapid onset of pain, frothy sputum and so on, you should suspect pulmonary embolus. If not, perform an ECG and look for tall 'peaked' P waves, which may give you an additional clue.

Other problems
On most occasions by now you will have a clear indication as to the cause for the patient's illness. If however, you have got to this stage and none of the foregoing conditions are apparent, it is worthwhile sitting down for a moment with the case notes (particularly if the patient's history is unfamiliar to you) and looking for additional problems that may cause the present situation. There are, as before, an endless number of these, but three at least should cross your mind, and these are:

- effects of drugs
- metabolic problems
- other illnesses.

Problems concerning drugs or medications that have been administered to the patient are almost endless. The patient may be allergic to, or having an adverse reaction to, a drug that has been prescribed. At this stage therefore you should look at the patient's chart, and consider in turn each of the drugs or medications being prescribed, and think about these points. In this connection, there is one particular group of drugs (steroids) that cause problems not infrequently after surgery, and for which you particularly should be on the look out. Steroids can affect the post-operative patient in a number of ways. First, they tend to retard wound healing, particularly if steroids have been taken for any length of time pre-operatively. Second, they tend to be associated with an increased predisposition to infection. Third, they tend to depress normal adrenal function. Generally this may not be a problem but, after the trauma of surgery, the dose of steroids may not have been increased sufficiently to deal with the effects of the operation. It is important in this respect to remember that the resultant clinical picture may range all the way from a full-blown Addisonian crisis to a minor problem. Indeed, I can remember encountering a whole range of patients whose post-operative vague problems were cured by increasing their dosage of steroids.

The next set of problems to look for are metabolic problems. In any appropriate textbook you will find descriptions of the symptoms and signs brought on by various metabolic problems following surgery. What the textbooks do not tell you, however, is that these symptoms and signs do not suddenly appear. Metabolic problems tend to 'creep up' on the patient, and they tend to surface most inopportunely at 3 a.m. in the morning when the hospital is least geared up to sort them out!

If you have got this far without uncovering the cause of the patient's problem, it is well worth sitting down for a moment with the input and output chart and the latest few sets of biochemical results. If you look for signs of over-or under-transfusion and study the last few electrolyte charts, you may well find something that helps you out of the dilemma. Naturally in an ideal world this should not be the case. The problem should have been detected and dealt with some time ago. Unfortunately however, there is very good evidence that this often does not happen. So, if you are still puzzled at this stage, a check of the last few days' biochemical and metabolic status may well be helpful.

Finally, while you are at this task, if the patient is not one whose background you know well, sit down with the case notes for a minute or two and look in the past medical history for a problem that might cause the present situation. Has the patient got a previous illness of which you are currently unaware, but that could be the cause of the current difficulty? It does not need to be added here that you look less than clever if the patient turns out to be a diabetic and you summon senior help to deal with a perfectly remedial hypoglycaemic attack. So, at this stage, study the case notes once again and review any previous problems that the patient has encountered.

Rule 4. Make a decision
In the previous paragraphs we have discussed some of the common problems and how to recognize them. In terms of managing the situation there is one final and important point that needs to be made. By now you should have recognized

the cause of the patient's problem and either treated it or you will have summoned help (e.g. if there is a major wound dehiscence). However, if by this time you are still sure that the patient is unwell, and you do not know why, *it is extreme folly to fall into the trap of waiting to see if the patient will get better*. Superficially, this is a very attractive course of action, but it is a poor decision nevertheless. If by this time (a) you are sure there is a problem and (b) you do not know what it is, you should be seeking help. In any case, you need to make a decision, and there are only three courses of action you can take:

- treat the problem
- go back to bed
- get help.

If you have already diagnosed the problem and can treat it, do so. If you are convinced the patient does not have a problem, leave well alone, but remember before leaving the ward to set parameters for calling you if things get worse. If you are still no wiser after covering all these aspects, at this stage you should be seeking help.

No senior colleague worth his or her salt, minds being called for a truly puzzling case. That is what they are there for, and that is what you (and they) owe to the patient. What senior colleagues *do* object to. is being called with some vague message, "Mrs. X isn't very well" and no details when they ask for them. That in turn is what you are there for. You may not be able to solve the problem, but if you go through the routine outlined in the previous paragraphs, at the very least you will have defined the problem. Then either get on with treating it, go back to bed, or get more experienced help.

8

Ethical problems in clinical decision making

So far in this book we have considered relatively clear-cut situations, even those where the evidence is finely balanced, and discussed how to proceed in a 'rational' or scientific manner in the patient's best interests. Indeed, many decision analysis experts proceed as if this is all there is to the matter. Anyone who has become involved in clinical medicine for any length of time knows that such a facile view is simply not true. As we have already stressed in previous chapters, it is indefensible to make a surgical decision if you have not already interviewed or examined the patient thoroughly, adequately and correctly, or indeed if you do not know enough medicine to know the risks and benefits of alternative forms of treatment. Sometimes however, this alone is not enough. There are situations and decisions where the eventual course of treatment is decided upon on the basis of issues that are neither scientific nor mathematical. Ethical problems occur because patients are people, often idiosyncratic or individual people, and for that matter the same applies to those responsible for their clinical care.

In days gone by, the Hippocratic oath formed the basis of medical ethics. Many of us from my own generation actually chanted the Hippocratic oath at the time of our graduation – luckily perhaps without realizing what we were doing. Looking back with 30 years hindsight I am slightly surprised to find that when I qualified I agreed not only to do my best for the patients, but to treat my teachers as my own parents, share my worldly goods with them, and even look upon their offspring as my own brothers!

Whilst one can only admire the basic ideas and principles behind the Hippocratic oath, much of it has been rendered inappropriate by the advent of modern medicine. For example, strict adherence to the Hippocratic oath would (amongst other things) prevent the keeping of case notes. The point is facile, but the implications are serious. Modern medicine has created a series of dilemmas and difficulties that are poorly understood, poorly taught, and sometimes not taught at all. They are often first encountered 'out of the blue' by the inexperienced doctor, and it is these ethical problems that probably cause more unhappiness and soul-searching than any other aspect of clinical practice.

In this chapter we are going to consider just a few of the ethical problems that can arise; and I am going to try and provide a framework for solving them, based chiefly upon a series of excellent seminars and workshops conducted by the Ethics Committee of the World Organization of Gastroenterology. In this way, even a small book such as this may help you to think the problems through clearly, and provide you with some comfort in what may be the most difficult situation you encounter in clinical medicine.

The human dimension to clinical decisions

At the outset, an important fact has to be faced. There is a major difference between a medical dilemma or decision and a similar dilemma or decision in many other scientific fields. It is simply this: in most other scientific fields the majority of decisions and dilemmas involve scientific and professional considerations but do not involve the scientist's humanity or attitude to society. Occasionally these attitudes may become caught up in scientific decisions, as with the development of nuclear weapons and so on, but in clinical medicine almost every decision or dilemma involves in some way the doctor's own humanity and the doctor's own attitude to society.

This is a proposition with which many of my own students have considerable difficulty. They have been educated, perhaps unfortunately, in their preclinical course to believe that they are becoming scientists and that the problems they will face and deal with are scientific problems. To be sure, I make no suggestion here that doctors or surgeons should proceed in an unscientific fashion. However, I do suggest that overlaying each medical decision is the doctor's own humanity and attitudes to society; and that in many surgical or medical decisions these attitudes come to assume increased importance, and sometimes dominate the decision. To explain this, consider the following example:

You are an ambulance driver with only limited paramedic experience. It is snowing and you are called to attend a major road traffic accident. Involved in the accident are two vehicles. The first is a Jaguar car and the second is a van with psychedelic graffiti on the side.

As you approach you notice that in the car are two middle-aged men in pinstripe suits, and you recognize, on the Jaguar, the parking badge from the consultants' car-park of your own hospital. In the van you can identify two twenty-year-old males with punk hairstyles and clothing.

All four of these people are badly injured. As far as you can determine they are all equally in need of immediate care and removal to hospital. Your ambulance however is only equipped to carry two people; and your assessment is that the two people you leave behind are more than likely to die.

Communications are out. No help is around. The two you take will live, those you leave will die. Which two people do you take?

Over the years, I have put this problem to successive generations of students. (You may care to make your own choice before reading further.) There are several types of response from most previous students. The response I personally like least is 'one of each'. This indicates those students with whom I am going to have difficulty later on to accept the need for taking decisions at all. However, when asked to choose between the two middle-aged men and the two occupants of the psychedelic van, the majority of students opt for the two middle-aged men. When pressed for a reason, they cite the possibility of dependant families, position in society and so on.

Relatively few students would take the two twenty-year old males (though one senior registrar said he would do so on the grounds he was due for promotion!). However, this is not all there is to the problem. There is a second part, which is only made known to the students after they have made their choice to the first part.

You now learn from bystanders and witnesses that the two gentlemen in the psychedelic van are members of the Salvation Army on the way to a charity concert with the 'Holy Rollers' Salvation Army pop group. The two middle-aged men in the Jaguar have stolen the car and are on the run from the police charged with embezzling hospital funds. Now which two do you take?

Now the overwhelming majority of respondents would choose the two young men. At this stage many students begin to argue. Some become quite annoyed. Some even claim the problem is unrealistic, and that in real-life one or other individual would have a *slightly* better chance of survival if left or taken and so on. In doing so, they have missed the point, which has nothing to do with the specific individuals involved. The point is simply to demonstrate that in many medical and surgical problems and dilemmas, it is the surgeon's or the doctor's own humanity and attitude to society that dominates the decision.

Of course this was an extreme example, but this type of problem and difficulty is found throughout surgical decision making; and unless you come to terms with this at a relatively early stage, the problems (if not the patients) will return to haunt you. In the remainder of this chapter we are therefore going to consider an individual patient, a specific example of a decision making situation that raises serious ethical problems. First, we will look at the situation itself, and next we will look at some ways of dealing with the situation, which help to clarify the issue and resolve the dilemma.

Sample case history

Let us consider how to deal with a patient where the principal problem in decision making is not so much logical,

scientific or surgical as one relating to ethics and management of an individual patient. The case history that follows
has been slightly altered (for reasons that will become clear
later) and is intended to illustrate some means by which you
can solve similar problems that will arise from time to time.
Note that as in previous chapters, we are not so much
interested in the precise details of the case as in showing you
a strategy that you can adopt in your own practice to solve
similar difficult cases. The case history now follows:

*An 80-year-old man is admitted to your hospital via the
Emergency Room with acute cardiac failure. His haemoglobin is 6.0/dl. and he has been passing tarry stools. He is
admitted to your surgical ward after stabilization with 2 units
of blood and appropriate treatment for his heart failure and is
in a stable condition. The reason for his surgical admission is
that rigid sigmoidoscopy performed in the Emergency Room
had demonstrated a large lesion, presumably neoplastic, at or
around the recto-sigmoid junction.*

*The records from the Emergency Room inform you that the
patient has been diagnosed (elsewhere) as having cancer, has
refused further investigation or treatment, and stated in the
Emergency Room that he did not want any surgery, any
'tubes', that he knew he was going to die, and wished to die
comfortably without suffering. Unfortunately, when you arrive to see the patient, he has become agitated and confused
and is refusing to take any nutrition. The family are present
and confirm only that the patient wishes to die comfortably.
They are unable to confirm the diagnosis, and you are unable
to ascertain where the diagnosis was made, or what the
original diagnosis was.*

*No one else is available for comment. How do you
proceed?*

If you have not already encountered a problem of this
nature, you soon will. If like most inexperienced surgeons,
you have not had to deal with the problem before, you will
find it difficult, and will be troubled by the implications of
the situation in which you find yourself. You may find it
helpful therefore to consider this sort of situation sooner

rather than later. As we discussed at the beginning of the chapter, this is a special situation, and one where in a sense there are no right and wrong solutions. Nevertheless, management has to be provided, you have to do something, and you may find it helpful to adopt the following strategy.

Step 1. Consider the options available

As we discussed in several earlier chapters, the first important step in any clinical decision making is to consider what options are available to you, and to consider the options from which you have to choose. So here, as in other situations, the first step in solving the patient's problem is to review those options and lines of management that you might possibly adopt. At least then you can be reasonably sure that you will not have missed out on an appropriate line of management by simply never considering it.

Table 8.1 lists a selection of possible options for the management of this particular patient's problem. These options represent a reasonable spectrum of possible modes of therapy. Notice that by listing them at this stage we do not necessarily endorse them or propose to follow them. We are merely listing the possible options so as to make an eventual choice after considering the case further.

Table 8.1 List of options of treatment for the patient described in the text

Euthanasia
Abandon all active treatment
Cease tube, relieve pain
Cease restraint
Maintain tube feeding
Substitute TPN + sedation
Resuscitate, investigate
Take to theatre

Step 2. Review the ethical principles

The next step before we discuss which particular option to adopt, is to review briefly some of the ethical principles that apply in this situation. This can be a lengthy and complex process (whole books have been written about biomedical ethics, and the interested reader is particularly referred to the excellent monograph by Beauchamp and Childress on the subject). However, for the purposes of our present discussion, there are perhaps four important ethical principles.

Beneficence

Doctors take on, both personally and professionally, a special obligation of beneficence to their patients. The Hippocratic oath states that "Into whatever houses I enter, I will go into them for the benefit of the sick", and even in this cynical day and age it is probably fair to say that a doctor who does not feel an underlying obligation of beneficence towards the patient has little place in medical practice.

There are, however, some problems with this admirable sentiment. One which does not particularly concern us here (but which will pose problems increasingly in the future) is beneficence to the patient versus beneficence to society, because it is not always appropriate or possible to do the best for each and every patient taking into account the need to allocate scarce resources. The problem that concerns us here is a more immediate one. It is all very well to say one will do what is 'right' for the patient, but in many cases it is difficult to decide what is 'right' for the patient, especially where (as in this case) the patient is no longer capable of rational evaluation of various modes of therapy.

Thus while the Hippocratic oath states "I will follow that system of regimen which, according to my ability and judgement, I consider for the benefit of my patients", this admirable declaration carries with it an implication ('Doctor knows best, dear'), which is increasingly unacceptable to the general public. Increasingly and probably rightly, the patient's wishes also count.

Non-maleficence

Again referring to the Hippocratic oath, the novice doctor declares that he or she will "abstain from whatever is deleterious and mischievous". Clearly this is fine in principle, in that the doctor's objective is obviously not to make mischief. (Later on the Romans got hold of this concept and translated into the aphorism *primum non nocere*.)

In the modern surgical world, we also have some problems with this part of the oath, because *primum non nocere* (above all, do no harm) has been aptly described as a nihilist's charter. Consider: if your objective is never to hurt the patient (which is what *primum non nocere* literally means) then technically speaking the surgeon would never take up a scalpel, nor would many other interventions such as therapeutic endoscopy ever be performed. The Hippocratic oath in this respect is unhelpful and the concept of *primum non nocere*, taken literally, has been rendered inappropriate by modern technically-based medicine.

How can this difficulty be resolved? Possibly here two considerations may help. First, instead of regarding the words *'primum non nocere'* in their strict or literal sense, it is helpful to regard this phrase as meaning 'above all do not do anything that will make matters worse than they are at present'. This actually comes very close to the original translation of the Hippocratic oath and (regarded in this light) the maxim *'primum non nocere'* is useful and helpful.

There is however a little more to it than this. In operating, or in performing an invasive investigation or intervention upon a patient, there is undoubted harm to the patient in the short-term (pain, disability, loss of earnings, or any combination). There is an absolutely crucial principle here, which was discussed earlier on p. 53. The reason that we are operating upon patients is because *despite the obvious harm in the short-term we do so in the expectation that the long-term benefits to the patient will outweigh the short-term harm.*

Non-maleficence is perhaps therefore best regarded as being a warning to all of us. As discussed in earlier chapters, the real problem for the surgeon is to evaluate the known harm done to the patient in the short-term by operative treatment against the expected long-term benefit to the patient in terms of the results of surgery.

Autonomy

As Gillon remarks, respect for *autonomy*, that is deliberate choice in areas of thought, will and action, is a central moral principle in a wide range of philosophies. Moreover, it is one that medicine has on the whole undervalued, as a result of its (understandable) concern for doing well for each and every patient with minimal harm.

Ideally, autonomy and the surgeon's respect for it, imply that a deliberate choice is made by a competent patient as to his or her management (on the basis of advice from the surgeon). This implies a number of principles; including a requirement for effective communication with the patients, telling them the truth, avoiding deceit, making efforts to discover how much information patients actually want, and attempting to provide them with this, and also attempting to discover the extent to which patients actually wish to be involved in the decision making about their medical care (and to cooperate with their wishes in this respect).

Problems start to occur when patients (for whatever reason) are less than fully competent to make such judgements. Perhaps the most common error in this respect is a belief on the part of many surgeons that impaired autonomy in a patient (the very sick, the very old, the confused and so on) means that respect for the patient's autonomy should be diminished or withdrawn. We all, unfortunately, are apt to fall into this trap in professional and private life. The classical 'give away' occurs when we start talking across elderly or frail patients or relatives as if they were not there, as in the famous phrase 'does he take sugar?' The point is extremely important. We have all seen situations where, in the presence of a confused or 'difficult' patient, the surgeon automatically takes over the role of decision maker and imposes his or her decisions upon the patient. We would all do well to remember that the impairment of a patient's competence should make us *more* (rather than less) considerate of the patient's autonomy, and *more* (rather than less) determined to find out what the patient's wishes were (or would be), and *more* (rather than less) willing to comply as best we can with them.

Justice

Justice, the final principle, is perhaps the most difficult of all to deal with, and has come to involve some of the most difficult decisions in clinical medicine. It implies three things. First, it implies a consideration of the laws of the land in which the doctor works. Second, it requires all people (not just surgeons) to treat each other fairly and respect each other's rights. However, third, the principle of justice requires a fair distribution of resources, and it is when these resources turn out to be inadequate to treat all patients optimally, that difficult dilemmas ensue.

I do not pretend to know the answer to such questions as what percentage of a country's Gross National Product should be devoted to health care. Nor do I pretend to know where the balance of responsibility lies for the provision of health care to an individual patient. I merely point out, with some sadness, the obvious. That there is not enough resource to go round, some form of rationing and prioritization system, which is both 'fair' and 'just' is desirable, and, most important of all, the medical education system, which encourages students to understand that everything can and must always be available for every patient, is imposing a cruel deception upon them.

To whom do these principles apply?

The easy answer is that all ethical principles outlined in the previous paragraphs apply to everybody. In the case of most patients it is not difficult to see that this should be so, but this principle is sometimes extremely difficult to apply in practice. For example, what about the comatose patient who cannot make his or her wishes clear? What about brain-dead patients? What about the embryo? What about the newly-born (badly deformed) infant? What about different kinds of animals? As Gillon points out, we may agree about all of the moral principles just outlined, but we might still disagree about the nature and moral status of special groups like those outlined above.

Gillon concludes his argument in delightful fashion by pointing out in the future there may even be problems about the moral status of very complex computers, or even extra-terrestrial beings! This leads to some delightful speculation – I will not add to it here, because I suspect that science fiction writers could do the concept more justice. But along with many others in the real world I regard the concept of diminished responsibility towards a patient because of their patient's diminished status as being highly dangerous practice. For the purposes of our present discussion I would argue strongly that the surgeon faced with *any patient* should consider the four overriding principles we have just discussed in deciding what to do for the best.

Step 3. Review of conflicts

The next step is to consider the possible options outlined in Step 1 and consider for each option the ethical principle discussed in Step 2. In doing so, each option should be assessed as to whether it conflicts with any or all of the ethical principles outlined. In this way, you may wish to eliminate some of the options, and thereby arrive at a short-list of one or two options, from which the eventual decision can be made. In the present instance some suggestions for this type of elimination process can be put forward.

Euthanasia is one possible option; but there are some heavy conflicts with several ethical principles. Euthanasia conflicts with the principle of non-maleficience, and in the UK at least it conflicts with justice, in that euthanasia is against the law of the land.

Cessation of therapy is also a dangerous concept. People often use the term but taken literally, it clearly conflicts with the principle of beneficence. What we really mean when we talk of cessation of therapy is the withdrawal of *active* or *curative* treatment and (most importantly) the *adjustment of management* to some other form of care. As Dunstan points out, we may properly withdraw active treatment when it is clearly ineffective; we may not withdraw therapy or medical care from the patient.

Operative treatment (at the other end of the scale) clearly conflicts with a number of ethical principles. It conflicts with autonomy as expressed by the patient, it conflicts with non-maleficence, and it also probably conflicts with some aspects of justice – in that scarce resource is being used to treat a patient who has requested treatment should not be given. (The same considerations probably apply to *invasive investigation*).

We have thus begun to narrow the options, because four of them clearly conflict with the ethical principles outlined earlier. In the middle range of management options, things become a little more difficult but nevertheless it is possible to treat these in the same fashion.

Restraining the patient also conflicts with both non-maleficence (in that the patient finds restraint hurtful) and autonomy (in that the patient does not want to be treated in this fashion). The same considerations moreover apply to *heavy sedation with maintenance of the previous regime*, particularly if this is compounded by feeding the patient through a nasogastric tube or even total parenteral nutrition. It is only too easy to argue that patients can be effectively and heavily sedated; but it should be remembered that this both conflicts with (to some extent) non-maleficence, and (to a considerable extent) with the patient's autonomy.

This leaves us with one final option *cessation of active therapy, relief of pain, and sedation*, and on the face of it this option would seem the best to pursue in the present instance. It is however, important not merely to make 'the right choice' (if there is such a thing) but to understand why one makes this choice. I personally have come across this sort of problem many times over the years, and I would probably make this particular choice. Why? Because it respects the patient's autonomy, because it is beneficial (in that it relieves pain and agitation), it does no harm to the patient, and there are no conflicts with justice.

You may find yourself in agreement with this course of treatment. On the other hand, since there is no right or wrong, you may feel that it is totally inappropriate and you may have alternative views. In the latter case, I would argue strongly that you are entitled to hold such views, but only if you have carefully and honestly reviewed all the options and only if you genuinely disagree with some of the remarks made in previous paragraphs. All too often this type of decision is made on the grounds of totally inadequate consideration either because the patient and relatives have not been consulted fully enough or (worse) 'because that is what we do here'.

Step 4. Make a decision

Once you have been through this process and narrowed your range of options, ruling out those that clearly conflict with various ethical principles, it is time to make a decision about the patient in question.

Ideally, such a decision should be made after close consultation with the patient. However, as in this present instance, it may not be possible; and if this is not so, you may wish to consult the relatives. Here there are some interesting differences across nations. In the UK, for example, it is common practice to discuss such a decision with the patient's 'next of kin', usually a spouse, or son or daughter. In other countries this is not necessarily true. In Eastern countries for example, it is customary for responsibility for the patient's welfare to be delegated not to a younger member of the family but to the head of the family, and it would be an unwise surgeon who ignored this traditional family procedure. In North America by contrast, some patients have delegated this responsibility legally by constructing a 'living will', and again it would be an unwise surgeon who failed to take this into account.

It is also worth pointing out that in selecting our chosen option for this particular patient we have chosen a course of treatment that will inevitably lead to the patient's early death. The difficulty here is that we strongly suspected (but did not know absolutely for certain) that the patient was suffering from a condition which was both malignant and incurable. This is perhaps the most difficult point to judge of all. I have argued (because I believe the evidence to be overwhelming) that the presumption of advanced malignancy was justified, and that further investigation of an invasive nature to establish this fact would not be justified. You yourself may well take a different view, and if you do, then it is my duty to respect your autonomy just as it is your duty to respect the patient's.

In doing so however, you would do well to remember the words of the Reverend Gordon Dunstan who remarked, "When a patient no longer expresses any interest in living further, and where the doctor agrees that the patient can have no longer an interest in living, then it is the doctor's duty to adjust the management to serve the patient's interest in dying".

Subsequent events

This was a real patient. Although this particular hospital was some way away I was asked to become involved in the problem and the management. On arrival at the hospital, the problem immediately became clear. In discussion, it emerged the patient (a general practitioner of 35 years standing) had known for some time of his condition and knew that he was going to die. He had, however, been given to understand (though not by the medical staff) that a signature on a consent form, consenting to 'whatever necessary', removed all his rights and privileges, and that an (unwanted) operation would be performed as soon as practicable.

Discussing the problem with the representative of the surgical team (who were incidentally completely blameless for this confusion) my immediate response was to proceed rapidly through the steps outlined and then suggest forcibly that 'when a patient can have no further interest in living, it is up to the medical team to serve that patient's interest in dying'. This was readily agreed, and the patient died the next day (of a concomitant massive cerebrovascular accident).

The patient was my father. Normally speaking it is not my practice to disclose patient names, and I do so here for two reasons. First, as a long-standing family doctor, it would have amused and comforted him to know that his difficulties might in the future years help others avoid inappropriate decisions. Second, it is important to emphasize how rapidly (after working through the steps outlined) an 'optimal' decision became apparent to all concerned. It is difficult to imagine a more stressful situation than recommendation of a line of therapy that inevitably will lead to the early death of one's own father. However, the steps outlined earlier made this relatively less painful and far easier for myself; and the next time you face a difficult surgical decision I suggest you adopt the same policy.

9

Putting it all together

So far, we have looked at several individual aspects of surgical decision making. We have studied decision making in its own right and we have looked at the applications of the principles of decision making to specific situations. Now the time has come to try and put all of these various pieces together.

In doing so, let us consider the progress of a young female patient with inflammatory bowel disease, from the first contact in the out-patients department, through admission for surgery, and until the complete resolution of her problems. In fact, it does not really matter which disease we consider, but inflammatory bowel disease is a good illustrative disease because many of the problems are complex and their management raises many of the issues we have been considering. We shall deal in turn with each encounter and discuss how to proceed in order to solve the patient's problems at that time. We begin as the patient walks through the door.

Initial out-patient attendance

You are a young member of the surgical team in the general surgical department of your hospital. You are on duty in out-patients, and have been asked to see new patients because the chief is away. Into your consulting room walks a young girl of 20. She has been referred to your out-patients by her family doctor and his letter is as illustrated in the Figure 9.1.

You interview and examine the young lady (see p. 12 for a suggested modus operandi) and confirm the findings in the family doctor's letter. You pay particular attention to abdo-

From: , MB ChB
Health Centre
Tel No:

12. sept 1989

To: Mr C
Consultant Surgeon
Dept of Gastro-enterology
hospital

Dear

Re: :22,

I should be most grateful if you would kindly see this young woman who complains of recent bowel upset. She was well till a week or so ago; but now complains of moderate diarrhoea (3 or 4 times/day) with rectal bleeding and also a little abdominal pain on defaecation. On examination, I can find little, but her Hb is only 12.1Gm/dL, and stool culture appears negative.

I wonder if she might have an early inflammatory bowel disease – possibly ulcerative colitis – and would be grateful for your opinion.

Thank you for seeing her

Yours sincerely

MB ChB

Figure 9.1 Initial letter from a family doctor referring a patient to the general surgical department with suspected inflammatory bowel disease.

minal and rectal examination where rigid sigmoidoscopy to 15 cm demonstrates a red and granular mucosa with some local contact bleeding and apparently continuous changes. How should you now proceed?

You should now proceed in the way that we have discussed in previous chapters and in principle the procedure is very simple:

- you need to *define the patient's problems* and what questions you need answered to solve them

- you need to *review the options available* to you and by a process of elimination, *select the preferred option*
- you need to *decide on what action is to be taken* to achieve your aims, treat the patient and manage the situation.

1. What is the problem?

The first thing to realize is the distinction between (a) the patient's problem and (b) your problem. The patient's problem is an attack of diarrhoea and rectal bleeding together with a little abdominal pain, which she would like addressed. Your problem is quite different. It is to provide answers to a series of very specific questions and it is these questions that dominate your thinking about managing the situation. In turn the questions you need to ask are as follows:

- has the patient got inflammatory bowel disease at all?
- if so, is it ulcerative colitis or Crohn's disease?
- what is the severity of disease?
- what is the extent of disease?
- are there other complicating factors affecting management?
- what is the appropriate management decision?

It is these questions that you need to be able to answer if you are to solve the patient's problem and manage the situation appropriately. Your actions therefore will be determined by the need to answer these questions. If you are able to answer them you will manage the situation correctly. If you are not, you will not manage the situation appropriately. So what you do is governed by the need to answer these questions.

2. What are your available options?

As in previous chapters, in attempting to manage the situation, the first thing to do is to review the options available to you. In the out-patients department, where you now find yourself, the options are a small and finite number along the following lines:

- return the patient to the family doctor
- do nothing but review the patient at a later date
- investigate the patient and review at a later date
- offer definitive treatment to the patient
- place the patient on the waiting list
- admit the patient urgently
- refer the patient to another speciality.

There may be other things that can be done with a patient in these circumstances, but not often and not many. So the first thing to do in deciding your course of action is to consider each of the above alternatives and decide which are reasonable for further consideration and which to rule out. In this way you may proceed quite rapidly towards deciding what should be the most appropriate treatment.

3. Selecting your preferred option

Let us first consider the various options and rule out those that are quite inappropriate. Option 1 (send away) is clearly inappropriate, because the family doctor referred the patient for your opinion and help. Equally inappropriate is option 2 (doing nothing), because the patient clearly has a problem and wants it solved. At the other end of the scale, you are not in a position to put the patient on the waiting list (option 5) because you do not yet know what the problem is and the patient may not in any case need admission to hospital. You are not in a position to admit urgently (option 6) because there is no indication to do so. To refer the patient elsewhere (option 7) would be an abrogation of your responsibilities, and to offer the patient definitive treatment (option 4) implies you know what the cause of the trouble is, and you do not yet know this.

The only remaining option is option 3, that of *investigating the patient*. Clearly at this stage this is how you should proceed. The patient warrants investigation, and on the other hand the patient is not sufficiently seriously ill to warrant admitting to hospital. Your selected option therefore is to investigate the patient and to ask her to return at an early date with the results of the investigations.

You may argue at this stage that you knew that anyway, and the clinically important problem is to decide which investigations should be performed. As regards the first point, the importance of the aspect lies not so much in selecting the right option as working through your options and excluding those that are inappropriate. Although in this case the option might be quite obvious, in many cases the option will not be so clear cut, and the *modus operandi* we have discussed is the best way to arrive at a sensible option.

As regards the investigations to perform, you may take the view that we have not already defined these. If so, you are in error. You have missed the point, because *we have already defined* which investigations need to be performed.

You may argue you never saw a list of investigations. True, there was none. Nevertheless, we still have defined what needs to be done. Remember the list of questions to be sorted out? *It is this list* that in turn defines which investigations to perform – these are, the investigations to answer the questions that we set out earlier (is it inflammatory bowel disease? is it ulcerative colitis or Crohn's disease? etc.).

Therefore, you will need to consider investigations to establish whether or not the patient has inflammatory bowel disease (e.g. stool culture if this has not yet been done). You will need to consider investigations designed to discriminate between ulcerative colitis and Crohn's disease (e.g. rigid sigmoidoscopy, rectal biopsy, barium studies, and possibly colonoscopy). You will also need to consider investigations designed to establish both the extent of disease (including the above radiological investigations) and also its severity. In this latter category for example, the famous Truelove and Witts severity scale includes such items as haemoglobin level and ESR, and so you will also need to get these investigations performed. Finally, you will need to consider other diseases and conditions that might interfere with, or affect, the management of the patient.

Therefore, your investigation list will finish up looking something like the investigation list in Figure 9.2. I repeat,

Has the patient inflammatory bowel disease?

stool culture

Is the problem ulcerative colitis or Crohn's disease?

rigid sigmoidoscopy
rectal biopsy
double contrast barium enema

How extensive is the disease?

(as above plus possibly)
colonoscopy
small bowel series
investigation of 'systemic' complications

How severe is the disease?

haemoglobin
white blood count
ESR
electrolytes, urea
serum protein levels
nutritional markers

Any other influencing factors?

depends upon patient history

Figure 9.2 List of possible investigations that might be performed. Note that far more important than precise investigations is the concept that each is performed in order to try and answer one of the specific questions raised. This list is not exhaustive.

however, that the precise investigations are not important. As we saw in earlier chapters, the important point is that each of your investigations should be for a purpose, and the purpose here is to answer one of the specific questions listed earlier.

4. Action to be taken

We have decided it would be appropriate to investigate the patient, and review her at an early date once these investigations have been performed. You may be tempted to surmise therefore, that the action to be taken is to investigate the patient and review in, say 2 weeks. If so you have never spent much time in the out-patients department. The action to be taken in order to answer the patient's problems is more than simply deciding to investigate the patient and review them at a later date. Specifically, there are a number of tasks that you need to perform. These are:

- you need to write up your investigational requests and make sure these are forwarded to the appropriate department
- you need to write up the patient's case notes in the way we discussed in Chapter 2
- you need to communicate this information to the patient's family doctor who referred the patient in the first place
- you need to talk to the patient, and tell her what your current thoughts are, what you are going to do to solve the problem, and where you and she go from here.

As regards writing investigational requests, we shall assume you know how to do this. I do urge you however, to read an article in the *British Medical Journal* (perhaps written with tongue in cheek) implying that biochemists are not gifted with ESP and suggesting that helpful referral notes are much appreciated. As regards your case notes and the letter to the doctor, you may care to have a look at the case notes in Figure 9.3 and the letter in Figure 9.4. These broadly speaking follow the guidelines we discussed in earlier chapters. They were generated by a computer; although you may feel you can add a human touch in your own notes and letters, if you cannot do as well as the concise, accurate, relevant notes in Figure 9.3 and Figure 9.4 you should think very hard about the notes and letters you are writing.

Finally, you need to talk to the patient remembering the difference between *information*, what you think you said, and *knowledge*, what the patient thinks you said, as discussed on p. 16. You need to inform the patient of your current thinking. You need to tell her what you propose to do in order to solve her problem, and where both of you go from here. You need moreover to do this in such a way as to

FIRST REFERRED ATTACK REPORT
PATIENT: HOSPITAL NUMBER:
SEEN BY: DATE:

PATIENT HISTORY:

Family History: Ulcerative colitis   Past History: Appendicitis
                   Tuberculosis   Fistulae

Smoking Habit: 10–19 cigarettes per day

Symptoms Began: September 1988   Normal Weight: 76 Kg

CLINICAL FINDINGS:

Weight: 60 kT   Pulse: 80 beats/minute   Temperature: 37.2°C

Bowels: Diarrhoea   Watery stools   8 bowel actions per day
                   No blood   Mucus+++

Pain: Mild   Colicky   Left Lower Quadrant

Tenderness: Moderate   Lower Half

Distension: Yes   *Nutrition:* good

Ano-rectal Exam: Fistula   *Digital Exam:* Pain

Sigy. Findings: Granular   Bleeding   Upper Limit: 15cms

Complications: Local   – enteric fistula
                   Systemic – jaundice

Other Abnormal Findings: Nil

INVESTIGATION RESULTS:

Radiology: (27th Jan 1989)
   Plain X-ray abdomen   Findings: Stenosis
                                                           Polyp

Biochemistry: (20th Jan 1989)
   Bilirubin   40 µmol/l

TREATMENT:
Prescribed in clinic:
      Asacol   150mg bd   One month
                   (then reduce to 50mg bd over two months)
Colifoam Enemas 1 per day   One month
                   (GP to continue this treatment thereafter)
Low residue diet

GP to prescribe:
   Salazopyrin   2 × 50mg tds   Three months

ASSESSMENT: Ulcerative colitis   Moderate

Figure 9.3 Sample set of case notes for patient with inflammatory bowel disease after initial encounter in the outpatients department.

Clinical Information Science Unit,
22, Hyde Terrace,
L E E D S,
West Yorkshire,
LS2 9LN.

Dr. A. Williams
The High Street
Fingalsham
Norfolk   2nd February, 1990.

Re: Linda SMITH   D.o.B. 28th Jan 1918
    101, Ledbury Road,   Hosp No 001
    Fingalsham,
    Norwich

Dear Dr. Williams,

I saw this patient, who suffers from Crohn's disease, at the clinic on 30th
January, 1990. The disease was moderately active, and she was having her
bowels open 3 times per day with right lower abdominal pain.

On ano-rectal examination, inspection showed no abnormality.

There was no local or systemic complications.

I have requested a double contrast barium enema, and blood has been taken
for the following investigations – haemoglobin, white blood cells, platelets,
potassium, chloride, creatinine, alkaline phosphatase, albumin and calcium.

I have prescribed a three months course of Prednisone, 10mg/day.

I will see her again in 3 months – though I would be happy to see her sooner
should you wish.

Yours sincerely,

Dr. A.T. Jones

Figure 9.4 Sample letter for patient in this situation (Note that Figure 9.3 and
9.4 do not refer to the patient discussed in the text. Figure 9.3 and 9.4 were
generated by computer.

bolster the patient's confidence, remembering the Lorentz
dictum that the patient attended your clinic in the hope that
you have seen this problem before and know how to deal
with it.

The one aspect that we have not dealt with so far concerns
the question of treatment. This is a matter of judgement. It

is perhaps a little premature to start offering specific drug therapy, remembering that you are still not sure the patient has inflammatory bowel disease; perhaps the best course of action is to suggest to the family doctor (e.g. in the letter) some symptomatic therapy, supplemented as soon as possible with specific therapy (e.g. Prednisolone 1 mg/kg daily in divided doses, up to a maximum of 60 mg daily supplemented by up to 4.8 g daily in divided doses, of your favourite 5–ASA drug), as soon as the investigational results confirm the presence of inflammatory bowel disease.

This is yet another reason why it is important to spend a little time talking to the patient. If the patient knows what you are recommending (and why) to the family doctor, the patient's trust will be maintained. Otherwise, the patient may believe the family doctor (who prescribes the treatment) is wonderful, but that idiot at the hospital did nothing.

Subsequent progress

Over the next few weeks, the investigations you ordered reveal a fairly extensive ulcerative colitis involving most of the colon. There is no evidence of Crohn's disease and no evidence of other complicating factors. The patient rapidly responds to the combination of steroid and 5–ASA therapy, and achieves clinical remission after a month. Over the next couple of years she is reviewed at increasing intervals in the out-patients department and has little in the way of further symptoms. You yourself leave the hospital and spend some time taking and passing relevant exams elsewhere.

Urgent admission to hospital

After a couple of years you return to the hospital, in a somewhat more senior position. Walking round the wards one day, you are surprised and disappointed to see the same patient back again. It transpires that she has been admitted to your ward following a referral to out-patients by her family doctor with a flare-up of her condition. The letter from the family doctor is shown in Figure 9.5 and represents on the

From: , MB ChB
Health Centre
Tel No:

11. Nov 1991

To: Mr C
Consultant Surgeon
Dept of Gastro-enterology
        hospital

Dear   ,

Re: :24,   .

This young woman has been under your care for ulcerative colitis for a
couple of years as an out-patient. You last saw her six months ago, at which
time she was well and in remission on maintainance sulphasalazine in a
dose of 1 Gm b.d.

She was well till 2 weeks ago; at which time she developed severe diarrhoea
(8–10 x per day) with frank blood p.r. and quite severe lower abdominal pain.
On examination today, she looks unwell. She has clearly lost some weight
and her Hb is under 10Gm/dL.

She is at present on oral steroids (prednisolone 20 mgm/day) as well as
sulphasalazine – but this attack appears quite severe. Perhaps you would
consider admitting her; and even the possibility of surgery if she does not
improve soon.

Thank you for seeing her, kind regards

Yours sincerely

MB ChB

Figure 9.5 Further letter from the family doctor requesting urgent admission for
a severe, acute episode.

*face of it a quite serious situation. The junior colleague who
saw the patient in the out-patients department felt it worthwhile (quite rightly) to admit her for your assessment on the
wards. Your interview and examination with her confirms the
details contained in the family doctor's letter. How do you
proceed now?*

You should by now know how to proceed. You should
proceed in the way we have discussed in previous chapters

and in principle the procedure is exactly the same as on p. 121, which is:

- you need to *define the patient's problems* and what questions you need answered to solve them
- you need to *review the options available* to you and by a process of elimination, *select the preferred option*
- you need to *decide on what action is to be taken* to achieve your aims, treat the patient and manage the situation.

1. What is the problem?

Once again the patient's problem and your problem are different. The patient's problem is that she feels unwell with severe diarrhoea, anaemia, lassitude, abdominal pain and general malaise, which she would like addressed. She is also apprehensive about the effects of possible surgery, and does not want it (especially an ileostomy) unless it is absolutely necessary. Your problem is once again to provide answers to specific questions, which will dominate your thinking about managing the patient. In this particular situation the questions are as follows:

- how severe is the patient's current disease?
- is her present conservative therapy adequate, or should it be amended in some way?
- what is the likely prognosis and what is the likely response to conservative therapy?
- should the patient undergo surgery? And if so, what kind of surgical procedure?

These are the questions that you need to be able to answer if you want to manage the situation appropriately. As before, if you answer them appropriately you will probably manage the situation correctly. If you do not, you probably will not.

2. What are the available options?

Next, you need to review the options available to you. If you do not consider them all, you may miss the correct management. As in the out-patients department, current options also are a small and finite number along the following lines:

- return the patient to the family doctor
- do nothing but review the patient at a later date
- investigate the patient and review after that
- as above, but institute intensive conservative management
- as above, plus prepare the patient physically and mentally for possible surgery
- proceed to operation immediately.

Possibly other things can be done in these circumstances, but not often and not many. So as before, in deciding your course of action each of the above alternatives should be considered and either confirmed as a reasonable course of action or rejected.

3. Selecting your preferred option

Of the various options we have listed some are clearly quite inappropriate. Sending the patient home (option 1) in these circumstances would be completely foolhardy, totally unwarranted and likely to cause harm to the patient. Equally, option 2 (doing nothing) is also totally unwarranted. This is not why the patient came to hospital. At the other end of the scale (option 6), whilst immediate operation may become necessary, you do not at this time have any definite evidence to warrant such a decision (though see below).

Of the remaining options, all are possible in theory. Clearly you will need information both from clinical observation and from special investigations (option 3) in order to assess the severity and extent of disease, and hence to infer the likely response to conservative management. Clearly also you will need to readjust the patient's conservative management (option 4) to take account of the new circumstances and increased severity of disease (remembering that the patient's conservative management not only involves increasing the dose of steroids and 5–ASA drugs but also possibly such measures as replenishing blood, iron, proteins, water and electrolytes, which may have become depleted as a result of the patient's severe bowel upset). Finally, you will also need (in view of the patient's stated preference for avoiding surgery) to prepare the patient both physically and mentally for a possible operation, which at the time of admission to hospital she regarded with some dread. The only option that fulfills these criteria is option 5 and clearly at this stage you should proceed with this option.

4. Action to be taken

As in the out-patients department, there are a number of tasks that you need to perform and a number of actions that you need to organize (even if you do not necessarily take all of them yourself). These include:

- you need to make it clear to all concerned (a) what information you want recorded about the patient, (b) what investigations you want performed, and (c) when you want these to be done
- you need to review the patient's biochemical, nutritional, and haematological status, and where appropriate institute supplementary therapy to restore each parameter to as near normality as possible
- you need to institute an intensive regime involving both systemic corticosteroids and oral 5–ASA drugs designed specifically to combat the patient's ulcerative colitis.

If you got as far as this and decided that you would institute each of these various actions, give yourself no more than two cheers, because there are some more actions that you need to take:

- you need to decide how long you will persist (if no improvement) before recommending surgery
- you need to make sure that the surgical team understand your criteria for abandoning conservative therapy and proceeding to immediate operation
- you need to ensure that the case records will be kept, to note relevant observations, so that you can be informed immediately if the patient's condition warrants immediate surgery

- you need to talk to the patient, tell her your current thoughts, what you propose to do to solve the problem, and where you and the patient go from here
- you need to consider the type of surgery and discuss this with the patient (you may, for example consider that colectomy and ileostomy would be preferable to procto-colectomy in view of the patient's views about ileostomy, allowing for a possible hook-up via ileoanal anastomosis at a later date)
- it may also be helpful in this connection for the patient to have a chat with another patient who has already under-gone the procedure in question, so that the patient can make an informed choice and feels involved in the process of management (the Ileostomy Association often have lists of volunteers whose services are invaluable in this respect)
- finally, you need to review once again the arrangements for supervision, and ensure that all those associated with management understand clearly (a) what observations are to be made, and (b) what are the criteria for calling you out with a view to considering emergency surgery.

Therefore, the decision to be made at this point is far from simple. Only when these aspects have all been considered, and the relevant actions have been taken to put your decisions into practice, are you entitled to feel that you have managed the situation in an appropriate way. Since, as we discussed earlier, it is uncertain now as to what will happen, there is nothing more for you to do at this stage except to sit back, watch carefully, and let nature take its course.

Subsequent progress

Five or six days pass without visible improvement in the patient's condition.

At the surgical unit ward round the patient is discussed fully and it is decided to proceed to surgery and to perform colectomy and ileostomy on the next operating list in a couple of days time. The patient has meanwhile had an opportunity to talk to an ileostomy patient and is much more reconciled to the procedure.

The decision to operate at this stage is actually clear-cut but it is worthwhile noting a few points, which refer back to the steps outlined in Chapter 6.

Step 1. The condition in which the patient finds herself is certainly one where surgery has a role to play. The patient's life is in danger, and she is in some pain. Surgery may help both problems. Therefore the first condition for surgery is already amply fulfilled.

Step 2. This particular patient also has a specific indication for consideration for surgery. The patient has a severe attack of disease. Conservative treatment has been tried over a period of a week, and she has failed to respond to this intensive period of treatment. There is, therefore, an indication for *urgent surgery* and an indication for the patient to be brought to the operating theatre on the next list.

Step 3. In this particular situation, experience worldwide shows that the 'risk-benefit' position has shifted quite dramatically over the last few days. The picture is outlined in Figure 9.6. If you want to construct a formal risk analysis table (see p. 53), by all means do so. The indication for surgery is, however, overwhelming in this instance.

Step 4. The choice of surgery is important. Colectomy and ileostomy is preferred to more extensive surgery (e.g. proctocolectomy involving removing the entire colon and rectum) for a number of reasons:

- it is a shorter procedure in an ill patient
- the risks of surgery are thereby lowered
- there is no perianal wound and recovery should be quicker
- it offers the prospect of further anastamosis and preservation of the anal sphincter at a later date
- it is the patient's informed choice.

Therefore, the decision to proceed to surgery, the timing of surgery, the operation selected all follow logically from the considerations we outlined in earlier chapters. The

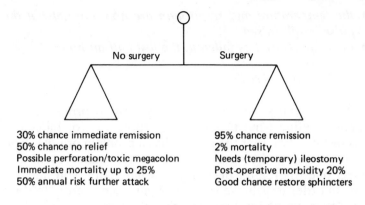

Figure 9.6 Risk-benefit analysis for a patient with a severe attack of ulcerative colitis. Note that in this situation, the balance is very firmly tilted in favour of immediate surgery. The mortality of surgery (2% in good hands, exemplified by large series from Leeds, Oxford, St Marks Hospital, in London, and other centres) is greatly outweighed by the immediate risk to life (25% in several series). For a further discussion see 'IBD some international data and reflections' (detailed reference in bibliography).

operation proceeds in routine fashion, the patient recovers from surgery and is making an uninterrupted recovery over the next 36 h.

Third Encounter – post-operative deterioration

It is 3 a.m. and you are woken by a telephone call from your junior surgeon on duty. The message you receive is along the following lines:

- *the patient is unwell and it is difficult to specify the reason*
- *the temperature, pulse and respiration are all raised*
- *the junior doctor found scattered wheezing on examining the chest and ordered physiotherapy*
- *this has been performed but the patient's condition has not improved*

- *the temperature and respiration are now normal but the pulse is still raised*
- *blood pressure has fallen in the last half an hour.*

How do you proceed?

By now you should know exactly how to proceed. You need to define what the patient's problem is (or indeed in this instance whether the patient has a problem or not). You need to review the options available for management and select one, thereafter deciding on what action you need to take in order to achieve your aims, and importantly to treat the whole patient and manage the situation.

1. What is the problem?

The 10–s check demonstrates that of the four categories listed in Chapter 7 (on p. 96) the patient clearly falls into the intermediate group. On the one hand the patient is neither dead nor moribund; but on the other hand the rise in pulse and respiration together with a fall in blood pressure strongly leads you to suspect that the patient *has* got a problem that needs sorting out. The question is, what is the problem, and what is your preferred option for dealing with it?

Cast your mind back to p. 96 in Chapter 7. First of all, what *type* of problem are you dealing with? Surely in this situation it is of the third type (serious problem, patient not moribund). This determines your preferred option, you cannot do nothing and go back to bed, you do not need to institute cardiopulmonary resuscitation measures, and the preferred option is clearly that outlined on p. 97 'serious problem – take it system by system'. That is your option, and that is the immediate action necessary.

2. Immediate action

A rapid repetition of the junior surgeon's examination reveals no evidence of external bleeding, a soft mobile abdomen with good bowel sounds, no stigmata of cardiac failure or focal weakness suggesting cerebrovascular accident, and a chest that is now clear following the physiotherapy. You know the patient's history well by now and there are no other diseases, such as diabetes, that might complicate the picture. The most recent haemotological and biochemical data give no particular reason to be alarmed.

Of course if your investigation had turned up some serious cause you would treat it. If the patient's wound was bleeding you would deal with this technical surgical problem, and so on. But this is not the case, or to be precise you have no evidence that it is the case in this instance. So whilst the scheme in Chapter 7 will enable you to take appropriate action 90% of the time, just for discussion let us imagine that this appears to be one of the other 10% of cases where you have to make an important decision under conditions of considerable uncertainty. This is a situation you will face from time to time. It is perhaps more worrying than all of the other situations put together and whilst neither this small book or any other comparable teaching can give you all the answers, perhaps some guidance can be given to help you through a most difficult time. How do you proceed?

You proceed as before, of course. You define the problem, list your options, select your preferred option, and take action. Here the problem is straightforward but difficult. The patient, 36 h after major abdominal surgery for ulcerative colitis is obviously unwell, but (probably) not due to one of the common post-operative complications involving operation, namely involving the cardiovascular or pulmonary systems. Your options are also fairly straightforward:

- go back to bed
- review in a few hours
- re-investigate in case you missed something
- consider other (rarer) causes
- return the patient to theatre
- ring the chief.

On the one hand you are, I trust, not proposing to take the patient back to theatre, because there is no real reason at the moment to suppose that this would be beneficial. On the other hand I trust that you are neither proposing to go back to bed nor (worse) to simply review the patient in a few hours time. (At least I hope not, because as we have pointed out elsewhere, putting off a decision is often tantamount to making no decision, and that is not what this book is about.) The same considerations apply to ringing the chief. You may need to, but perhaps not quite yet.

Two other options are open to you. First, you can think about re-examining and investigating the patient in case your initial impression has missed something. Second, you can ask yourself whether there are any causes that *might* be responsible and which are amenable to treatment without much risk or harm to the patient. Actually neither of these options are mutually exclusive. So it might be as well to proceed with them both while monitoring the patient's condition. Therefore, an ECG and chest X-ray might just help; as may a rapid haematocrit and repeat serum electrolytes and urea. All simple investigations, rapidly done, but may help you to be more confident in ruling out some of the common causes.

There is however, one condition we have not so far considered, that often presents in an insidious fashion and which is readily amenable to treatment. Maybe you have already worked out what it is, if not, reference to pp. 97 to 102 might refresh your memory.

A bolus injection of 100 mg of hydrocortisone hemisuccinate is drawn up and you administer this intravenously yourself. Within 5 min the patient's condition has reverted to normal.

On the ward round next morning you remind your junior staff (who are suitably impressed) that any patient who has been on steroid therapy for any length of time may (even though the operation is covered by increased dosage of steroids) require quite substantial enhancement of the steroid dose to cope with the trauma of the immediate post-operative period. If you are wise however, you will also remind yourself that the only reason you managed to think clearly at 3 a.m. in a difficult situation is that you followed carefully the scheme set out in Chapter 7.

Subsequent progress

Ten days later, after an uneventful post-operative course, the patient is discharged from hospital and some time later undergoes a successful ileoanal anastomosis. Time passes by and a year or two later you are accosted in the street by a delightful looking young lady whom you do not recognize but who greets you warmly and thanks you for being so wonderful. Your wife, who is accompanying you, raises her eyebrows at your protestations of ignorance and innocence, and only after considerable thought do you recognize your former patient now restored to health and vigour.

Leeds is a relatively small town, and I have to admit that this latter situation used to happen to me occasionally. How you deal with this problem is up to you. Speaking personally my own long-suffering wife believed me, so I cannot help you with sound advice concerning this last problem; except the consoling thought that at least you know you have made some good surgical decisions, and you can further console yourself with the additional thought that it is better to have a living problem than a dead certainty.

10

Twenty-first century medicine

The hard-pressed medical student or junior surgeon, after a busy day on the wards or in the operating theatre, may be forgiven for taking the view that the main objective is to get through the week, never mind about worrying what is going to happen in the next century. I know the feeling well. If you feel this way, I sympathize. Nevertheless, there are some reasons why, in a quiet moment, you would find it helpful to sit down and think about twenty-first century medicine, and as time goes by you may well be increasingly glad that you did.

The first fact to be acknowledged is that any student entering clinical medical school at this time will be unlikely to practice medicine independently this century. If you think about it, and add up 3 years in a clinical medical school as an undergraduate, 1 year pre-registration, and 3 or 4 years before higher certification, this takes the student up to the end of the century before post-vocational training is complete.

There is a second reason why you will need to consider twenty-first century medicine right now. If you look back to Chapter 1, remember the imperatives set out there. The medical course is finite, teachers are becoming increasingly busy, and the amount for a student to learn has exploded. These trends are going to accelerate if anything, and by the beginning of the next century the traditional methods of learning surgery will have become totally inappropriate if you are to keep up with current trends. Clearly therefore, you need to think now about the future if you are to get the maximum benefit from your present undergraduate and postgraduate courses.

A third reason why you need to consider the twenty-first century is that constant change is taking place and the situation in the next century is likely to be quite different from that at the present time. This applies to techniques of surgery. Already many of the surgical techniques, which I learnt laboriously in the 1960s, are no longer practised to any great extent. Perhaps the most important change however, is the advent of information technology. As we saw earlier, wisely used this can help greatly but like everything else information technology is open to abuse, and you need to be familiar with its strengths and limitations if you are to practise medicine and surgery effectively for the rest of your career.

Perhaps the most important reason why you need to consider the next century however, concerns an aspect already touched on, that is to enable you to make the best possible use of your present course. I personally know of no curriculum that actively sets out to teach medicine and surgery appropriate for the next century. There have been suggestions that *every* curriculum *should* do so; but such changes take time, and it would surprise me if twenty-first century medicine was actually taught before the twenty-first century came along.

If you are lucky, your curriculum will prepare you for clinical practice in the 1990s. If you are not so lucky you will wade through a curriculum designed in the 1960s only to find at the end of that time that most of what you have learnt in that time is of very little use in your day to day practice. If so, you can at least minimize the ill-effects of this by going through the curriculum with your eyes open, picking out those aspects that are particularly likely to be important in your future practice, and paying relatively less attention to those that are not.

In order to do so, however, you need to think a little bit about the twenty-first century and which aspects and skills are likely to be desirable, so that you can concentrate upon these. In the remainder of this chapter, therefore, we are going to consider a few aspects of twenty-first century medicine, a few of the problems, and a few of the topics and skills on which it is desirable to concentrate during your training period, so as to enable you to take good decisions during your future career and future surgical practice.

Important aspects of twenty-first century medicine

1. The scope of medicine

At the risk of becoming repetitious let me remind you of what was said in Chapter 1, because it stands at the heart of all that we shall do in the next century. It is no longer possible to know the whole of medicine. By the end of the century it will no longer be possible to know the whole of surgery, or even (I suspect) to know everything there is to know about a surgical speciality or particular topic. If you go through your training period with the aim in mind of 'knowing everything there is to know' about your chosen speciality, you are likely to be disappointed. If on the other hand you go through your training period realizing that encyclopaedic knowledge is impossible, you will be more likely to learn thoroughly the important basic knowledge, you will make better use of your training, and you will make better decisions in the future.

2. What you need to be able to do

Of course the surgeon in the twenty-first century will need to have the same skills in handling tissue and the same detailed knowledge of operative technique. These will depend upon your chosen speciality, and also upon the operations in fashion at the time, and clearly a detailed description is out of place (and indeed impossible here).

Already however, some authorities have been looking forward to the next century. In a fascinating series of articles in the *British Medical Journal*, Don Berwick, A Enthoven and John Bunker have listed what they describe as "new clinical skills" of modern medical care. These include:

- awareness of interdependence
- ability to work in teams
- ability to understand work as 'process'
- skill in collecting, aggregating, analysing and displaying clinical data
- skill in designing health-care practices
- skill in collaborative exchange with patients
- skill in working collaboratively with lay managers.

I am not sure I agree entirely with everything in this series of articles (though I urge you to read them), but the authors certainly have a point when they argue that new skills are going to be needed; and some of these (4 and 6 on the list above) may sound familiar to you by now. One problem however, with their list is that they do not spell out the clinical side of the list; so let us consider that aspect further. In addition to the managerial skills, therefore, there are some clinically orientated core skills that you will need to acquire, and the most important of these are:

- cardiopulmonary resuscitation
- ability to communicate
- core knowledge
- how to access unknown information.

The first of these is vital. It is in my judgement quite scandalous that members of the medical profession (in whatever speciality) often have very little knowledge of modern techniques of *cardiopulmonary resuscitation*. When they come across an accident or a major medical emergency, they have less idea sometimes of what to do than informed bystanders. This is totally unacceptable; and so the first skill you will need to possess, and constantly to practise, is the ability to perform cardiopulmonary resuscitation.

It is also true that whatever speciality you finally finish up in, you will need *the ability to communicate with patients*. Here I agree with Berwick and colleagues. If you cannot communicate effectively with patients and with colleagues you are likely to be in difficulties whatever your precise speciality – and we discussed some of these aspects in Chapter 2. The implication of this is clear. You should constantly 'throughout your course' take every opportunity to communicate with patients, with colleagues and with friends, and practise your skills consciously so that when the time comes you will be an effective communicator. Remember that the commonest complaint amongst patients (whether or not litigation is involved) is that they were not kept in the picture. In the future, with the increasing complexity of medicine, communication is likely to become increasingly important.

The third aspect, *core knowledge*, is clearly important. Obviously, the doctor or surgeon who does not have basic biomedical or clinical information (as we discussed in Chapter 2), or the doctor who lacks basic medical information, is a menace on the wards or in surgery, and should not be permitted to practise. There is however one further aspect of this, which you would do well to think about during your course. This concerns information regarding *health care delivery systems*. Again I agree with Berwick, Enthoven and Bunker, and it is quite clear from present trends that the surgeon, like every other doctor, is going to be increasingly involved in complicated teams of health-care workers and in complicated health-care delivery systems. You would do well to remember as you go through your course that somewhere and somehow you are going to need to pick up information about these health-care delivery systems and in particular the one in which you work, if you are to make maximum and effective use of it.

The final desirable skill is important, for two reasons. First it is likely to be increasingly relevant during the next century and second, it is virtually untaught in most medical curricula. This skill concerns the *accessing of unknown information*. It applies to clinical information, it applies to administrative information, and as we discussed earlier, it may save you from the dilemmas caused by the explosion of knowledge. To repeat, the effective surgeon in the next century is not going to be the surgeon who 'knows it all' but rather the surgeon who has a sound core knowledge and who knows how and where to access all the information that is not readily at the finger-tips.

3. What information can be accessed?

Obviously at this point we enter the realms of speculation, or as I would prefer to put it, the realms of informed prediction based upon the projection of current trends. As we discussed earlier, information technology is currently in its infancy, but already it seems reasonable to suggest that by the end of this century many of the current pioneer schemes and systems will have become universal practice. The surgeon or physician in clinical practice at the end of the century might therefore reasonably expect to have some form of access system to information concerning the various aspects of medicine set out in Figure 10.1.

The table lists a number of aspects and broadly these can be grouped into three categories. First, *administrative information*. This is already available in many hospitals, but unfortunately since the systems have largely been designed by administrators, they tend at the moment to provide information useful to administrators and not to doctors. It is already possible to see this trend changing, and by the end of this century useful information concerning the logistics of clinical practice will be readily available to surgeons in two respects. One, the current administrative situation will be available upon request – for example the bed state, the patient load, the work-load of the unit, and so on. Two, information concerning other parts of the health-care delivery system will be available so that, for example, a surgeon who wishes to refer a patient to a particular hospital can readily access information that will describe the situation in the unit or hospital concerned. There may even be 'league tables' so that a surgeon with a particular problem can refer the patient to the 'best available specialist', but this at the moment is highly debatable.

The next aspect of information, which is already becoming available, concerns *information regarding the particular patient facing the surgeon*. Several attempts have been made

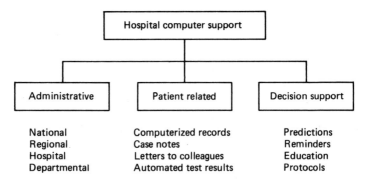

Figure 10.1 Types of hospital computer support.

since the 1960s to computerize the patient record. Most of these have been an outstanding failure; but the more recent systems are beginning (belatedly) to demonstrate at least some practical value. All sorts of problems have occurred, and many others have been raised (such as security and so on), to delay the introduction of the paperless department. Personally, I cannot wait for its introduction, which I think will occur first, particularly, in specialized departments. Computers and information technology are by no means infallible. But when one considers that 10% of case notes are unavailable when they are needed (and when one considers the rapidly increasing mobility of patients and doctors), the computerized patient record has much to commend it, provided the early mistakes and difficulties can be avoided and overcome.

The third and final aspect of information access in the twenty-first century is both the most difficult and the most exciting. This concerns *decision support*. Again many mistakes have been made. In the early 1960s there was talk of computers taking over from doctors and even talk of the 'post-doctor era'. All of this was extremely foolish and set the field back for decades. It is however, clear, for the reasons already mentioned, that some form of help is needed and systems are now emerging, which increasingly in the future will become both necessary and effective in providing the sort of help we need to counter the information explosion.

In speaking of 'decision support' we therefore mean a variety of systems designed to help the doctor or surgeon make more effective decisions. There are many ways in which this can be done and it is difficult to predict which one or more of these will eventually prove most effective and acceptable. Minimum datasets (such as we discussed in Chapter 2, Chapter 3 and Chapter 5) have much to commend them. Diagnostic suggestions based on the sort of decision analysis we discussed in Chapter 4, may prove increasingly valuable, though here I suspect that suggestions rather than probabilities will be more acceptable and easier to handle. Suggestions concerning treatment might also be acceptable, though here again I suspect that surgeons will not take kindly to being told what to do by a computer. Far more likely to be acceptable are indications of prognosis (e.g. with treatment A, the patient has a 40% chance of recovery, whereas with treatment B, the chance is 70%).

4. Computer power versus human reason

In previous chapters and paragraphs, we have seen that medicine is developing at such a rate that the human mind is increasingly incapable of keeping up. We have discussed in previous chapters some ways in which you can minimize the problem. We have in this chapter suggested that in future, computers may do much to help. Therefore it becomes relevant in the last paragraphs of this book to consider the role of surgeons and computers in the next century.

The title of this heading 'computers versus humans' is deliberately provocative, because that way lies disaster. The only answer I can see is some kind of 'symbiotic' relationship between the two. As a surgeon in the future, if you rely entirely on your own ability to reason, retain and remember, you will increasingly become ineffective. As a surgeon in the future, if conversely you rely entirely upon the power of the computer to store and retrieve information, you will also become a liability. The only future salvation that is likely to be effective is to make the best of both worlds – using the computer's power to store and retrieve information, and blending this effectively with your own humanity and ability to reason.

We have not yet done this well in medicine. We are much less advanced than other industries (e.g. the aircraft industry) where a lot of these problems have been tackled and have been to a large extent overcome. You might argue that medicine is difficult and different. We have disposed of that argument earlier. You might argue that human life is too important to be left to a computer. You might even believe this to be true; but there are some interesting consequences. For example, the next time you travel by air, as you come in to land in thick cloud, as the wheels go down and you still cannot see the ground, if you truly believe that human life is too important to be left to a computer, now is a good time to get out and walk.

One final thought. One of the reasons why the aircraft industry has so successfully blended computers and humans is that the people involved heavily in the design of the systems were themselves pilots, practising their art on a day to day basis and at the same time designing systems to improve it. The same applies clearly in surgery and in medicine generally; there is an equal need for practising surgeons to become involved in the design of systems that aim to help them in the twenty-first century. If this is not done we shall see systems emerging whose aims and construction are totally foreign to surgeons. They will not be used, and if they are used they will not be effective.

This would be fine except for one thing. The imperatives we discussed in Chapter 1 will not go away. Failure to take on board the changing demands and opportunities of new technology can only (inevitably) widen the gap between efficacy (what *can* be achieved) and efficiency (what *is* actually achieved).

The solution, in principle, is simple. Surgeons of the future need to be involved in these new technologies, helping with design, evaluation, implementation and ensuring that such systems are clinically relevant, useful, and up-to-date. I hope that amongst this band of future technocrat surgeons will be some of those who have read this book. If so, I wish them luck. The task will not be easy, though the rewards will be great; but then come to think of it, this is true for the whole of surgery as well.

Further reading

Early on in the book, I pointed out that there was a quite massive literature concerning decision making and clinical practice. I also emphasized that much of this literature was totally inappropriate for the average medical student or clinician. There are however, some books and series of articles that are favourites of mine, which can be understood by non-mathematicians (on the principle that if I can understand them, so can most non-mathematicians!) and might be helpful and interesting to readers of this book who want to progress further.

In discussing them I have not followed traditional practice. Instead of merely listing the references I have grouped them under a series of topic headings and tried to say a little bit about each so that if you wish to pick a specific reference you can hopefully find the one best tailored to your needs.

General

Davis P J and Hersch R (1980). *Descartes' dream: the world according to mathematics*. Brighton: Harvester Press

When I was sent this book for review, I thought someone at the *British Medical Journal* was joking. How wrong I was! If you thought numbers and mathematics were dull, read this book. If you want to know the answers to such questions as 'are we drowning in digits?', 'can love be computerized?', or 'are we hooked on unreasonable but effective computers?', read this book. If you do read the book, and still think numbers are dull, there is not much more that I (or I suspect anyone else) can do about it.

Wulff H R (1976). *Rational diagnosis and treatment.* Oxford: Blackwell

Professor Henrik Wulff is a genial, pipe-smoking philosopher thinly disguised as a leading Danish gastroenterologist. If the first few chapters of the present book have caused you to wonder exactly what diagnosis is all about, Henrik Wulff's book will repay further study. In particular if you now wonder why we are burdened by such terms as 'so and so's syndrome' when we really do not know what we are talking about, read Henrik Wulff's book and find out who is to blame for this muddle.

McClachlan G, ed. (1976). *A question of quality: roads to assurance in medical care.* Oxford: University Press

In the last few years we have all become almost obsessed with questions of quality. Some people talk about audit, some about quality assurance, some about quality control, and so on. There have been quite a few textbooks on the subject; but none better than this early example of a collection of essays on the topic of '*quality of health-care*'. None are better than this early collection of essays by giants in the field. You may have difficulty getting hold of a copy but if you can it is worth reading. If you cannot secure a copy or if your library cannot provide it, you may care to know there is a new journal out entitled '*Quality in Health Care*'. The first few issues contain some excellent articles and if this is your interest, I suggest you either subscribe or get your library to do so.

Troidl H, Spitzer W O, McPeek B *et al.* eds (1986). *Principles and practice of research: strategies for surgical investigators.* Berlin: Springer Verlag

I selected this book for further reading because of the breadth of issues that it tackles. As well as the usual titles such as 'some things you should know about computers', there is a wealth of information for students and young surgeons on how to go about surgical research (e.g ten tips on preparing research protocols, ethical principles in surgical research, how to appraise published research, and so on). A most rewarding read.

Decision making

Lusted L B (1968). *Introduction to medical decision making.* Springfield: C. C. Thomas

During his formative years, Professor Lee Lusted was radiologist in Chicago, and when he turned his attention to clinical decision making he brought to the subject both the commonsense and objectivity that many radiologists possess. This is a superb book and although it has been around for some time, I really do not think that anything better has been written on the subject. It covers all of the issues in Chapters 2 to 5 and provides the interested reader with a great deal of information on these subjects.

Lindley D V (1971). *Making decisions.* London: Wiley Interscience

This is another small volume written 20 years ago about decision making which I think has not been bettered in the last couple of decades. When he wrote the book, Dennis Lindley was Professor of Statistics at University College, London, but please do not let that put you off! There are certainly some mathematical equations in the book, but there are also quotations from authors ranging from Shakespeare to Bertrand Russell, and even quotes from the Guardian newspaper! Great Fun!

Galen R S and Gambino S R (1975). *Beyond normality. The predictive value and efficiency of medical diagnosis.* New York: John Wiley

If I had my way, every medical student would be forced to read this textbook and be examined in it before being let loose on patients. What this book deals with, purely and simply, is the value of special investigations in predicting the diagnosis. My own firm belief is that no doctor should ever write up a patient for a test (see p. 22) unless the doctor knows the value of the test, and this is quite simply the best textbook in this area.

X   Clarke J R (1990). A tutorial series on surgical decision making. *Theoretical Surgery*; **5**: 105–6,129–32,206–10 and (1991) **6**: 45–51, 110–15, 166–76, 177–83

If you wish to read something further specifically related to surgical decision making, you cannot do better than to get hold of (if you can) this tutorial series on surgical decision making by John Clarke who is Consultant in Charge of the Emergency Room in the Medical College of Pennsylvania in Philadelphia. John Clarke (with various co-authors) deals with such vital topics as diagnostic accuracy, probability, test results, resolving trade-offs, patient attitudes, and so on. Your library may not take the journal concerned, but it is well worth trying to get hold of copies of these excellent articles.

Clinical topics

Cope Z (1991). *Early diagnosis of acute abdomen*. 18th Edn. Oxford: University Press

Chapter 5 is all about the acute abdomen, and Zachary Cope's textbook (which first came out in 1923) is the definitive textbook on the subject. The fact that it is now in its 18th edition speaks for itself. (There is even an edition in verse, 'The Acute Abdomen in Rhyme!' which Zachary Cope wrote under the *nom de plume* of 'Zeta').

de Dombal F T (1991). *Diagnosis of acute abdominal pain*. 2nd Edn. Edinburgh: Churchill Livingstone

Modesty forbids me to say too much about this small volume, but whereas Zachary Cope's definitive textbook is all about one person's experience, this volume is drawn on data from over 50 000 patients around the world. Perhaps the two complement each other, and after reading both you should know something about the acute abdomen.

de Dombal F T, Bouchier I A D, Myren J, and Watkinson G, ed. (1982). *Inflammatory bowel disease: some international data and reflections*. Oxford: University Press

Just as Zachary Cope, and my own textbook in Chapter 5, give you a background to the acute abdomen, the collected reflections of the World Organization of Gastroenterology Council and Survey Team should give you a similar background into the world of inflammatory bowel disease. This may be helpful to read in conjunction with Chapter 9.

Ethics

Beauchamp and Childress (1983). *Principles of biomedical ethics*. 2nd Edn. Oxford: University Press

This is an excellent foundation if you wish to know more about biomedical ethics. Other possible avenues that you might care to explore include the specific issues of ethics in gastroenterology published by the World Organization of Gastroenterology Ethics Committee, and you might care also to follow up specific matters by referring to the *Journal of Medical Ethics*, which should be in most libraries.

Future issues

If like me, you are worried about where we are going in the future and would like to think about twenty-first century medicine, there are a number of entertaining publications that would repay reading.

Kleinmuntz B (1990). Why we still use our heads instead of formulas. *Psychology Bulletin*; **107**: 296–310

You may have wondered after reading some of the issues in Chapters 3 and 4 why we still bother to go on using our heads instead of mathematics. Ben Kleinmuntz would agree with you, and has produced one of the most entertaining discussions of the subject I have read for many years.

Berwick D M, Enthoven A, and Bunker J P (1992). Quality management in the NHS. *British Medical Journal*; **304**: 235–98 and 304–9

I selected these articles, partly because they are from the *British Medical Journal* and therefore easy to get hold of, but mostly because they deal with absolutely crucial issues for the future in terms of quality management and what skills you will need to possess in the next century in order to function effectively. A most thought provoking series of articles, these are an excellent follow-up to John Bunker's earlier book (Bunker J P, Barnes J A, and Mosteller F (1977). *Costs risks and benefits of surgery*. New York: Oxford University Press, which deals with many of the issues we have already discussed in Chapters 2, 3 and 4 and in particular in considering the decision to operate. Both the articles and the book are warmly recommended.

Journal of Medical Education (1984). Publication of the Association of American Medical Colleges. Part 2. 1–200

Finally, if you want to know what is happening or likely to happen in medical education in the next century, this thought-provoking series of recommendations should be of considerable interest. You may be pleased to see some of the recommendations ('medical students should have less facts crammed down their throat!'), and you may be less pleased with other recommendations ('medical students should know about information technology'). You cannot fail however, to be stimulated by the report; and it is difficult to read this report without realizing just what changes are going to be needed to function effectively in the future.

Index